China's Health Situation, Policy, and Law

www.royalcollins.com

China's Health Situation, Policy, and Law

Wang Yue

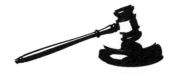

Books Beyond Boundaries

ROYAL COLLINS

China's Health Situation, Policy, and Law

Wang Yue

First published in 2024 by Royal Collins Publishing Group Inc.
Groupe Publication Royal Collins Inc.
550-555 boul. René-Lévesque O Montréal (Québec)
H2Z1B1 Canada

ISBN: 978-1-4878-1278-2

To find out more about our publications,
please visit www.royalcollins.com.

Contents

Historical Evolution and Prospect of Medical Law in China

I. Introduction of Medical Law Concepts

The term "medical law," originating in Japan and Taiwan, China, has only recently come into use in mainland China. Its connotations and extensions were not well defined domestically by the time of introduction, winding up a relatively vague and ambiguous concept. Judging from this stage, the academic community's use of medical law is still quite confusing.

British scholar Morgan believes that medical law is a response and that whether it is an independent discipline no longer matters. If medical law is a hybrid, it includes contract law, tort law, and criminal law, at least administrative law, procedural law, trust law, conflict of law, labor law, and now it is more clear; it also includes some aspects of personal and intellectual property law.

In Japan, medical-related laws are summed up as the "medical affairs law," with the most representative books such as *Medical Law* and *Medical Dispute Prevention Law—Medical Affairs Law* by Professor Tetsu Ueki as an example. These works focus on the law centered on the handling and adjustment of medical disputes and explain the comprehensive medical affairs law of medical law research. It can be seen from this that the medical affairs law discussed by Japanese scholars mainly refers to the regulation of medical disputes and legal relationships caused by medical acts. Its meaning and extension is medical law, which adjusts legal relationships related to medical practices. As far as legal elements are concerned, medical law is part of health law. The connotation and extension of traditional health law are broader than medical law. Therefore, medical law should refer to the general name of laws and regulations that mainly regulate the legal relationship of medical services in health law.

II. Awakening of Patients' Rights Awareness Has Made Medical Law Explicit

The healthcare industry has long been a secluded kingdom running its own rules of the game. The law rarely intervenes in medical industry affairs. The public trusts this discipline, and physicians treat patients with the same respect as teachers, as Hippocrates required. Naturally, this means medical personnel are not the target of expensive and potentially destructive lawsuits. Therefore, judges have also, to a large extent, allowed physicians to set their own industry standards and conduct collective professional evaluations as long as the standards are widely accepted by peers. This approach may not keep the standards at a very high level; it may only be the minimum level that can be tolerated. However, this concept means that it is difficult for patients to prove that physicians' negligence is responsible; what is even more frightening is that the medical industry lacks the motivation to continuously improve and improve itself. Facts have shown that this attitude of high autonomy in the medical industry does not always set very high industry standards; on the contrary, it may simply be basic and not in line with the intention of national health policy, that is, the standard of best interest to patients. I recently saw the Indian Medical Association (IMA) claim that 75% of physicians will experience physical or verbal violence during their careers. This statistic is surprisingly similar to 59.79% of physicians experiencing physical or verbal violence in the White Paper on the Practice Status of Chinese Physicians published by the Chinese Medical Doctors Association in 2014. This is clearly not a coincidence but rather a law of social development. No matter what country it is, along with social progress and an increase in citizens' education level, the police society will inevitably evolve into a civil society, and the awakening of people's sense of rights will become a common characteristic of all progressive societies. This is bound to question, challenge, and even resist traditional healthcare industry culture. For example, two of the three major human rights movements that marked the evolution of modern American culture, namely the women's rights protection movement (such as discussing the legalization of abortion), the minority rights protection movement (such as the anti-discrimination campaign for black Americans), and the patient rights protection movement, are all closely related to the medical community, as can be seen.

The 40 years of reform and opening-up witnessed booming growth in all walks of life, yet bringing forth concerning issues therefrom. For a long time, physicians have helped the world with the mentality of "treating the disease like a family member," and patients have also often been rewarded with a sense of gratitude for "a present-day Hua Tuo" and "kindness and benevolence." The doctor-patient relationship is extremely harmonious. However, with the development of China's market economy, the doctor-patient relationship in the past has changed. Moreover, the physician-patient sides have turned against each other and gone to court. The change in the doctor-patient relationship is not due to changes in the biological attributes of patients who are the recipients of medical services but rather because their social attributes have changed dramatically. The most typical sign is the awakening and expansion of patients' sense of rights. This requires that medical school students, as future doctors, must have a clear insight into this change and understand that medicine is not only a "benevolent art" but also a "human art."

Medicine and law are two very different disciplines and majors, but since these two majors are research on "people," they are bound to be closely linked. In particular, with the continuous improvement of laws and the increasing awareness of individual rights in society, legal issues related to medical practices will inevitably become a hot topic and focus of common concern for the public and medical community. As a medical professional who meets the requirements of modern society, he must find a balance between saving the world and saving lives and his legal responsibilities. He must re-understand many basic concepts in medical-legal relationships. However, traditional medical education in China often ignores the cultivation of humanities and social science literacy, making it impossible for medical personnel to meet social development needs. Along with the awakening of patients' rights and the increase in doctor-patient disputes, the legal rules for handling medical disputes have gradually become obvious science, which is a matter of concern for the medical industry and the legal community.

III. "Patient-Centrism" Trend in Medical Law Legislation and Judiciary

1. Looking at the trend of "patient-centrism" from changes in standards for judging medical negligence

> *Medical negligence as defined in the Measures for the Handling of Medical Accidents*

Article 2 of the 1987 Measures for the Handling of Medical Accidents stipulates that the subjective fault of the subject of medical accidents is "due to negligence in diagnosis, treatment, and nursing care." In 1988, the Ministry of Health's Explanation on Several Issues Concerning the Measures for Handling Medical Accidents divided diagnosis, treatment, and nursing errors into careless and overconfident errors. It stated that "to constitute medical accident negligence, it must be illegal and harmful. Illegality: In a medical accident, it mainly refers to a violation of the rules, regulations, and technical operation procedures for diagnosis, treatment, and nursing. These can be written, or they can be conventions that everyone follows in practice." Medical negligence, as defined in the Measures for the Handling of Medical Accidents, only refers to "negligence in diagnosis, treatment, and nursing," and the corresponding judgment standard is "diagnosis, treatment, and nursing standards and practices."

In the process of drafting the 2002 Regulations on the Handling of Medical Accidents, the judicial authorities pointed out that "medical treatment and nursing regulations" were insufficient to cover all medical negligence. If medical personnel did not even fulfill their general legal obligations with respect to the rights and interests of others stipulated by law, then their actions were clearly gross negligence. The drafting authority drew the above opinions, so it revised the criteria for judging medical negligence of medical institutions and medical personnel to read: "Medical and health manage-ment laws, administrative regulations, departmental regulations, and diag-nosis, treatment and nursing standards and regulations."

> *Medical negligence as defined by the Tort Liability Act*

In the civil law community in China, although there is a difference between the "three elements statement" and the "four elements statement" about the constituent elements of the tort, both statements acknowledge that fault is a necessary element for the composition of a tort act. Except for a few scholars who insist that fault is an act and an objective concept, the vast majority of scholars believe that fault, in terms of its attributes, is a subjective psycho-logical state of a person and, therefore, a subjective concept. Scholars still insist that fault is a concept that combines subjective and objective factors. Although the mainstream view holds that fault is a subjective concept, the criteria for judging fault show an objective trend. The so-called fault stan-dard refers to what is used to judge whether the infringer was at fault when committing the infringement. British tort law uses "the degree of care that should be achieved" as the standard for fault judgment. In theory, the "level of attention that should be achieved" also has a dispute between "subjec-tive standard statement" and "objective standard statement." The "subjective standard statement" determines whether there is a fault by judging the in-fringer's state of mind. The "objective standard theory," which now occupies the mainstream view, is to compare the infringer's behavior through some kind of objective behavior standard and to infer whether there is any fault in the subjective aspect of the infringer's behavior from the external manifesta-tions and characteristics.

After the formal implementation of the 2010 Tort Liability Act, how to understand the "failure to fulfill the duty of diagnosis and treatment corre-sponding to the medical level at that time" referred to in Article 57 of the Tort Liability Law of the People's Republic of China (hereinafter referred to as the Tort Liability Law) is a very important issue. Wang Shengming, a major participant in the Tort Liability Law, believes that fulfilling the ob-ligation of diagnosis and treatment referred to in Section 57 includes, of course, the requirements of laws, administrative regulations, regulations, and medical regulations. However, the medical staff fully complied with the above requirements, and there is still a possibility of fault. The key question is whether other medical personnel generally make this kind of mistake. A similar view also argues that, under normal circumstances, medical personnel can fulfill their obligation to avoid harm to patients through careful action or inaction. There are also opinions that the duty of care is the most basic obligation of medical personnel. In the process of providing medical services to patients, medical personnel are required to do their best to be careful and concerned about patients, so as to protect the lives and health of patients from harm other than the permissibility of medical treatment. Scholars believe that the duty of care of medical personnel includes the duty of care in general and the duty of special care. The former includes the obligation that legally practicing physicians should pay attention to, while the latter includes the obligation to explain, inform, refer to a doctor, consult a doctor, and observe and care. Other scholars believe that medical personnel are obligated to pay close attention during medical activities. It is commonly believed that the duty of high care is a higher duty of care than that of a good manager. Some scholars suggest that "the level of medical care at the time" is not equal to the "level of medicine at the time" and that regional factors should be taken into account. "The level of medical care at the time" and the former is not an abstract concept; it must include the two dimensions of breadth and depth. Breadth is the question of the scope of the duty of care under the medical standards at the time; depth is the question of the extent to which the duty of care must be achieved under the medical standards at the time.

From a comparative legal point of view, objectification of fault judgment criteria has indeed been the development trend of tort law since the 20th century, that is, starting from the need to protect victims, reducing the burden of proof on victims, making it easier for judges to judge faults, thus better serving the need for accountability. Therefore, Tort Liability Law adopts the "objective standard" theory in the fault standard. The "objective standard" is proposed as a "good father" standard in civil law and a "rational person" standard in English and American law. This kind of legal fiction is not the "highest standard of conduct," nor the "general standard," but the "above average" standard, that is, the standard of conduct of a reasonable and prudent person.

> ### *Legislation will accelerate the shift from "physician-centrism" to "patient-centrism"*

In fact, the current clinical situation in China is very similar to that of Britain 30 years ago. The phenomenon of physicians not paying attention to respecting patients' autonomy is very common in clinical practice and medical research. The idea that patients have the right to make their own decisions is often drowned in the rampant paternalism in the healthcare industry. Today, the mainstream slogan in the UK is no longer "Physicians Know You Best." "Doctor-patient partnership" is the slogan preferred by the current British government. To ensure patients' best interests, the generally accepted principle is that physicians should negotiate rather than be arbitrary. This shift in ethical views is most clearly reflected in current industry and legal regulations, which require informed consent from patients who have the power to decide. Industry-specific regulations As the General Medical Council claims: "A successful doctor-patient relationship is built on trust. To build trust, patients' autonomy must be respected—it is up to them to decide whether to carry out a medical intervention ... They must be provided with sufficient information in a way they can understand to enable them to make informed medical decisions."

Just as the doctor will not simply think that what the physician is doing is correct and then win the case simply because of the view of "acting responsibly," the patient will also not simply think that what the physician is doing is incorrect and then win the case simply because of the view of "acting responsibly." In both cases, although the viewpoint of "responsible peers" is important, this viewpoint is not automatically equivalent to a legal conclusion. The judge has the power to identify and review the testimony of "responsible peers." Obviously, the shift from "patriarchy" to "patient-centrism" from experts and witnesses monopolizing factual determination and judges meddling in factual determination all made the medical industry feel very dissatisfied and difficult. Because litigation undoubtedly has a strong deterrent effect, making those working in clinical settings always vigilant.

2. Looking at the trend of "patient-centrism" from unaware patient agency system changes in emergency treatment

> *Era of "agents for family members, agencies, and related persons"*

The Hospital Work System promulgated by the Ministry of Health in 1982 includes regulations on surgical signatures in its operating room work system. However, it does not stipulate that patients have the right to make their own decisions; the exact opposite is the rule. Before surgery is performed, the patient's family or patient unit must sign and agree. At the same time, it also stipulates that body surface surgery may not be signed by the family or unit. In the case of emergency surgery, if it is too late for the medical staff to obtain the consent of the family or agency, the patient's attending physician may sign and be carried out with the approval of the department director, director, or business deputy director.

Section 33 of the Regulations on the Administration of Medical Institutions promulgated by the State Council in 1994 actually made some refinements and improvements on the basis of the above regulations, and stipulated that the right to decide on surgery, special examinations, and special treatment was divided into three situations: in the first case, if the patient is conscious and can express opinions, the patient's consent must be obtained, and the consent and signature of the family or related person should be obtained; in the second situation, if the patient's opinion cannot be obtained, the consent and signature of the family or related person should be obtained; in the third situation, if the patient's opinions cannot be obtained and no family or related person is present, Or when other special circumstances are encountered, the attending physician shall propose a medical treatment plan and implement it after obtaining approval from the head of the medical institution or the person authorized to be responsible.

In this era, the author summarizes it as the "patient and family or related person sign" era, which means that the patient's right to make independent decisions is not confirmed by law in China. Instead, in addition to the patient's consent, the consent of the patient's family or related person (such as the unit) must also be obtained. This is clearly contrary to the basic spirit of patient autonomy and self-determination. However, in the era of "unit people," although this provision is unsatisfactory, it must also have its helplessness.

> ### *Era of "family agency"*

The Law of the People's Republic of China on Medical Practitioners, promulgated by the Standing Committee of the National People's Congress in 1999, stipulates in Section 26 that physicians should truthfully introduce the condition to patients or their families, and that carrying out experimental clinical treatment should be approved by the hospital and obtain the consent of the patient himself or his family. Although the text uses the description of "patients or their family members," the author believes that this is the first time that China has truly established the legal status of patients' right to make independent decisions in legislation. According to the explanation of the Interpretation of the Medical Practitioner Law of the People's Republic of China jointly prepared by the National Office of the Legal Affairs Committee of the Standing Committee of the National People's Congress, the Department of Policy and Regulation of the Ministry of Health, and the Department of Medical Administration of the Ministry of Health, in medical activities, physicians and patients are both people with independent personalities. Still, there is a clear difference due to their different levels of medical knowledge. Physicians have an active advantage. Facing patients are often in a passive acceptance position. Physicians take initiative over the patient's health condition and should make the best choice to relieve the patient's pain, but they should not lose their independent status as a result. On the premise that treatment is not affected, physicians should respect the patient's wishes and truthfully tell patients about the condition during the disease diagnosis and treatment process, so that patients can promptly understand information on diagnosis, treatment, prognosis, etc. so that they can exercise their corresponding rights to the diagnosis and treatment of the disease. Only when the patient is incapable of acting should he truthfully introduce the condition to his family, which is regarded as an extension of the patient's ability to make decisions independently. However, lawmakers still have a strong "good father" scenario. For example, they emphasize that under the premise of the patient's informed consent, purely technical decisions should generally be based on the physician's opinion. Still, issues involving personal lifestyles and attitudes should respect the patient's wishes. If breast cancer patients know their condition honestly, they can make a decision to remove all of the breasts to prolong life or remove part of the mass to maintain a good body shape.

The Regulations on the Handling of Medical Accidents promulgated by the State Council in 2002 actually continued the provisions of the Law on Practicing Physicians, that is, medical staff should truthfully inform the patient of the patient's condition, medical measures, medical risks, etc., and answer his or her inquiries promptly.

> ### *Era of "close family agency"*

Articles 55 and 56 of the Tort Liability Law in 2010 mark the evolution of China's patients' right to make independent decisions from the era of "patient or family signature" to the era of "patient or close family signature." First, the Tort Liability Law abolishes the use of "family members." In fact, "family" is not a strict legal term. It generally refers to family members other than yourself within the family. Its extension is vague and unclear, and in practice, it is easy to cause differences in understanding. Secondly, the Tort Liability Law chooses "close relatives" in legal terms. In commonly used legal terms, "immediate blood relatives," "side blood relatives," and "close relatives" are all used. For example, China's Marriage Law uses "immediate blood relatives" and "collateral blood relatives" within three generations. However, it is clear that the extension of "immediate blood relatives" and "collateral blood relatives" is not suitable for actual clinical use. Hence, the Tort Liability Law finally determined that "close relatives" were used.

"Close relatives" in China's laws have different meanings in different legal departments. The meaning of "close family" in civil law and administrative law is the same. They all refer to spouses, parents, children, siblings, grandparents, grandparents, grandchildren, and grandchildren; however, the scope of "close relatives" in criminal lawsuits is smaller; it only includes husband, wife, father, mother, child, woman, and siblings.

> ### *What has never changed is the "undercover agent"*

The "undercover agent" referred to here means that if a patient is unconscious in emergency treatment and has special circumstances (for example, family, related persons, or close relatives cannot be contacted, etc.), the law designates who will act on the patient's behalf to make independent decisions, to make clinical decisions that are most beneficial to the patient. In reality, from the Hospital Work System to the Regulations on the Administration of Medical Institutions to the Tort Liability Law, although the range of agents that are often preferred for patients who are unaware (their families, related persons, or close relatives) has changed, the above legal systems have all set "undercover agents" for unaware patient agents under special circumstances in emergency treatment: that is, medical institutions.

> *From "physician-centrism" to "patient-centrism"*

The Hospital Work System promulgated by the Ministry of Health in 1982 and the Regulations on the Administration of Medical Institutions of the State Council in 1994 do not specify that patients have the right to make their own decisions but instead stipulate that the consent and signature of the patient's family or unit (person concerned) must also be obtained. This legislative consideration is not only related to the social and historical background at that time, but also how to determine the agent who is in the best interests of the patient when the patient is unconscious. The wider the scope, the more convenient it is for the doctor's work, so it can be called the "physician center doctrine." In 1999, starting from the Licensing Physician Law, China truly established the system of patients' autonomy in decision-making and no longer allowed the patient unit (related party) to act as an agent for the patient's best interests; further, in 2010, agents with the best interests of patients were reduced from family members to close relatives. It may be inconvenient for physicians' work. Still, narrowing the scope of agents is undoubtedly more beneficial to surrogate opinions close to the patient's own expression, so it can be called "patient centrism."

IV. Alienation and Solution of Medical Law in Medical Institutions

Over the years, hospitals have often simply "treated the symptoms" and punished doctor-patient disputes. It even distorts "medical ethics" with the idea of "negative protection" in order to reduce immediate disputes. Not long ago, I discovered at a tertiary hospital that the "Surgical Consent Form" had been renamed the "Surgical Volunteer Form." If you take a closer look at the patient signature column, almost all of them start with the words "request," "require removal of the ovaries on both sides," and "require platelet transfusion." Hospitals have more exemptions of all kinds that need to be signed and texted in medical-legal documents, yet one finds that physicians are less and less informed about the various risks in the documents. As a result, we hope to eliminate liability and reduce disputes through medical-legal documents. Yet, there are more and more disputes and complaints, which are not even resolved through legal means, but rather seeking self-help relief. This is a clear phenomenon of "alienation." In particular, when doctor-patient disputes are frequent, it seems that such "medical treatment" can act as a kind of "negative protection" for doctors. Soon, you will discover that "volunteer books" and "requests" do not relieve medical personnel of their legal responsibilities to patients; instead, they will make the doctor-patient relationship antagonistic, alienated, and even apathetic; you will find that this kind of "negative protection" will cause the phenomenon of misuse of tests and shamming of critically ill patients over and over again, and eventually lead to both physicians' and patients' losses.

If you are a current clinical medical staff member, what kind of occupations do you usually dislike the most? They will tell you in unison: "Teachers, lawyers, journalists, civil servants, and doctors." Yes, these five types of "learning patients" often make medical staff angry, because they have a strong desire to know and a strong ability to seek knowledge. We shouldn't be complaining and blaming, because what's the point of complaining and blaming? As society develops, you will find that more and more patients are joining the ranks of learning patients. Patients can use their mobile phones to search for medical expertise outside the clinic. The Internet has ended the era where medical personnel monopolized expertise. But our medical staff are still used to the "patriarchal doctor-patient relationship" (For your own good, listen to me, don't ask so many questions, just do what I say). However, the "patriarchal doctor-patient relationship" is actually over; only a "friend-style doctor-patient relationship" (based on shared learning and discussion) can satisfy the "learning patient." Legally, the "informed consent" system does not affect protecting medical personnel. Yet, today, the vast majority of clinicians still understand it as "exemption from liability," "protecting doctors," or "going through a procedure" and "burden" Few medical personnel have raised "informed consent" to the level of educating patients to view and pay attention to it. This is also the reason why we have made patients sign more and more disputes over the years. Looking forward to the development direction of medicine internationally, in the face of "learning patients," foreign medical staff choose "active change": using multimedia courseware, VCR recordings, and App applications to significantly reduce workload while improving the ability to educate patients. However, our domestic medical staff still complains and blames patients for their increasingly demanding and difficult-to-serve ...

If we want to improve the doctor-patient relationship, we must first let physicians know that our interests and those of patients are unified because today's doctors will also become patients tomorrow. What rules and attitudes we use to treat patients today will be what rules and attitudes we follow when we welcome our parents, children, and colleagues tomorrow. Second, physicians should be made to understand that the cornerstone of maintaining a doctor-patient legal relationship is trust, and that trusting relationships must adhere to the basic principle of "putting the other party's interests first"; otherwise, they cannot win the other party's trust and trust. Physicians must overcome "delicate egoism." Third, physicians should be made to understand patients' rights, because if a person's biological attributes are reflected in every cell, then a person's social attributes are reflected in every right. As long as you respect every patient's right, professional risks for physicians will be minimized.

Medical Justice

I. Concept of Medical Justice

Justice has always been regarded as a virtue and a lofty ideal in human society. Justice is considered an age-old concept in both China and the West, but there is still no consensus on what justice is. Edgar Bodenheimer states, "Justice has a protean face, capable of change, readily assuming different shapes, and endowed with highly variable features. When we look deeply into this face, trying to unravel the secrets hidden behind its outward appearance, bewilderment is apt to befall us."[1] It is perhaps for this reason that justice has fascinated numerous thinkers, at all times and in all countries, with its appealing charms. To this day, it still attracts many thinkers to try to unravel its mystery. The theories of justice of Domitius Ulpianus, Plato, and Aristotle are different, but all have the basic connotation of "giving everyone what he deserves." Marcus Tullius Cicero also described justice as "the spiritual orientation of mankind to give everyone what he deserves."[2]

It can be seen that justice is the highest category of legitimacy, reasonableness, and fairness, and its basic connotation is to grant everyone what he or she deserves.[3] Justice is an eternal value ideal pursued by human society. Throughout human history, thinkers have devised a variety of ideal models

---

1   Edgar Bodenheimer, *Jurisprudence: The Philosophy and Method of the Law* (Beijing: China University of Political Science and Law Press, 2004).

2   Aristotle, *The Politics* (Baltimore: 1972), Book I, Chapter 2.

3   Aristotle, *The Politics* (Beijing: The Commercial Press, 1997).

of a just society. From Plato's The Republic in ancient Greece to St. Thomas More's Utopia in modern times, from the society of great harmony and unity in ancient China to the harmonious society of socialism in contemporary China, all of them reveal the people's pursuit of an ideal society of justice in different eras.[1]

The concept of justice and its connotations seem to be interpreted differently across academic areas. In the field of jurisprudence, justice may well be understood as the supreme value of law.[2] However, there is still no consensus among legal researchers on the interpretation of the types, functions, and connotations of justice.[3] As one of the legal orders, the medical order should also follow medical justice to guarantee the protection of human rights in medicine. As far as medicine is concerned, the sense of justice is a feeling of medical morality, which is specifically manifested in the medical staff's courage to redress the balance in medical activities and insist on the dignity of human life.[4] From a legal point of view, the author describes medical justice as including the right of all citizens to enjoy reasonable medical resources in a medical society on an equal basis. Moreover, the people should have the right to participate in deciding how to utilize and allocate medical resources. Human rights in medicine should be guaranteed in terms of the attribution of responsibilities arising from medical activities.

II. Equity in Medical Services

Due to the limited medical resources and the differences in individual needs, people are forced to seek relevant principles to effectively allocate medical resources under the premise of a reasonable medical burden, so as to reconcile the possible conflict between the right to life and the right to

---

1 John Bordley Rawls, *A Theory of Justice* (Beijing: China Social Sciences Press, 1988).

2 Arthur Kaufmann, *Rechtsphilosophie*, 1997, S. 152.

3 Reinhold Zippelius, *Rechtsphilosophie*, 1994, S. 200ff; Kurt Seelmann, *Rechtsphilosophie*, 1994, S. 125ff. In this paper, it is argued that the legal order should comply with the requirements of the concept of justice.

4 Tse Bosheng, "Introduction to Medicine: Series of Medical Humanities II" (School of Medicine, National Taiwan University, 1997).

equality. The distribution of healthcare resources involves the contest of political power. When civil society and civil organizations desire to have more resources allocated to them, the question of justice will be addressed. From the perspective of society as a whole, how to distribute resources in a way that is more in line with the principles of fairness and justice should be a topic that will be discussed for a long time in China. It can be concluded that health and medical care, as well as social welfare, must be the issues of the utmost importance in contemporary China.

Equity in healthcare means that every citizen has equal access to the healthcare services he or she deserves when he or she needs them, so that he or she can meet the basic standard of living. It is mainly manifested in the reasonableness of the allocation of medical service products in any area and among any population group, as well as the reasonableness of people's access to basic medical services. Equity in medical services in China is mainly characterized by the level of medical service financing and the provision of medical services.

1. Financing of medical services

The allocation of medical resources can be divided into three levels: the first is the political level, which determines the proportion of the total national production to be allocated to the medical and healthcare sector; the second is the medical level, which determines the most important medical services (in the order of priority); and the third is the patients' level, which determines the patients who should be provided with special medical services. These three levels are not independent, and each higher level restricts the choices at the lower level. The social resources allocated to the medical and healthcare sectors affect the range of services available and the rigor of patient selection. Decisions at the patient level also affect the choices made at higher allocation levels, resulting in a tightening of funds for other healthcare items.[1]

---

1 Ezekiel Emanuel, ed., *Medical Ethics in End-of-Life Care*, trans. Liu Lizhen (Taiwan: Wu-Nan Book Inc., 1999).

From the structure of China's total health expenditure, there is indeed a shortage of financial input. Both the proportion of total health expenditure and its share in fiscal expenditure are on a downward trend and are relatively low even when compared with those of developing countries. According to estimates, the proportion of government health investment in total social health expenditure dropped from 23% in 1991 to 15% in 2001. The proportion of residents' personal health expenditures increased from 39% to 61% during this period. The proportion of the government's expenditure on health to the state financial expenditure during the 6th Five-Year Plan period was 3.1%, but by 2001, it had dropped to 1.7%. With China's economic development, national expenditures on health and other social services have not risen, but have instead declined. It is obviously the precondition for the difficulties in access to healthcare. For this reason, it is necessary to increase financial investment in healthcare, improve the urban and rural medical security system, and broaden the scope of medical insurance coverage.

2. Utilization of medical services

At present, the utilization of medical services in China is not equitable in general. It manifests itself in insufficient fairness in the allocation, accessibility, affordability, rationality, and quality of the utilization of medical and healthcare services.[1]

(1) Allocation of medical resources. In marked contrast to the government's insufficient investment in healthcare, a large number of medical resources are currently lying idle in China. It is understood that, at present, nearly 70% of the primary and secondary hospitals in China are in a state of loss. In other words, on the one hand, the bed utilization rate of large hospitals can be as high as about 110%, while on the other hand, that of small hospitals is only about 36%. Doctors in China receive about 4.5 consultations per capita per day, while many doctors in large hospitals receive more than 60 consultations per day. In fact, there are quite a large number of doctors in China. In 2000, the number of doctors per 1,000 residents in

---

1   Shi Li, Zhang Kaining, and Jiang Runsheng, "Discussion on the Theoretical Framework of Equity of Health Service," *Chinese Health Service Management*, no. 1 (2003).

China was 1.67, which is close to that of the United Kingdom and Japan. Therefore, while people complain that it is difficult to receive medical treatment, a great number of medical and healthcare resources remain unutilized in primary and secondary hospitals. The distribution of healthcare resources is highly unbalanced throughout the country.

The Primary Health Care Law of the People's Republic of China (hereinafter referred to as the Primary Health Care Law), which is being drafted, must balance the country's healthcare resources. First of all, the National People's Congress should define in the law a reasonable ratio of government health investment to GNP and a reasonable ratio of government health investment to total national health expenditure. Secondly, the National People's Congress should make it clear at the legal level that the government's investment in healthcare must be tilted towards economically underdeveloped areas, so as to alleviate the imbalance of medical and healthcare resources between regions in China. At the same time, the Primary Health Care Law should clarify the system of hospitals for first diagnosis in order to resolve the imbalanced distribution of medical and healthcare resources among hospitals at all levels in cities. The hospital of first diagnosis means that patients who receive medical treatment at public expense and those who are insured by urban medical insurance may choose different hospitals of first diagnosis depending on the types of illnesses they suffer from. It should be specified in the legislation that only primary hospitals or community hospitals should be the first choice for common and chronic diseases. If grassroots hospitals are unable to provide treatment, a referral system should be strictly implemented in accordance with the Regulations on the Administration of Medical Institutions.

(2) Accessibility of medical services. The current social medical insurance system has a narrow coverage, covering only all urban employers in China, including enterprises, government agencies, public institutions, social organizations, private non-enterprise units, and their employees. Rural areas remain a "blind spot." As of the end of October 2002, a basic medical insurance system had been established in 98 percent of the country's integrated areas, covering a population of 86.91 million, less than 1/13 of the

total population. The majority of the population, especially rural residents, are not covered by medical insurance.[1]

The government must strive to provide "basic medical care for all." On the basis of the scale of the existing basic medical insurance system, the government should expand the coverage of medical insurance for social groups through policy support and guidance and increase the coverage of social security programs for social groups, especially disadvantaged groups. Since it is not yet possible to implement a social health insurance system in rural areas, the government should actively develop a rural health security mechanism that combines cooperative medical care and government subsidies.

(3) Affordability of medical services. Due to the regional differences in economic development in the current market economy, the population's income level is polarized, and there is a large gap between the rich and the poor. The demand for medical services is multilayered and diversified. High-income earners have excessive access to healthcare services. On the other hand, those with low incomes have to pay too much out-of-pocket medical expenses as a proportion of their incomes and are even unable to receive basic medical care services. As a result, there are cases where people become poor due to illness.

The government should expand the coverage of social medical insurance and actively develop a multi-level medical insurance system founded on basic medical insurance. On this basis, it should establish and perfect a social medical assistance system and intensify its efforts to assist the impoverished through multiple funding sources and multiple levels of contribution standards and entitlements.

(4) With regard to the quality of medical resources utilization, due to regional and temporal differences in economic development, the quality of medical services varies among social groups who pay the same medical fees at different times and in different regions. It is mainly characterized by differences in service technology, service attitude, and the skill level of service providers. That is to say, it cannot meet the uniformity requirement of medical commodities.

---

1   Chen Yingyao, Wang Liji, and Wang Hua, "Evaluation of Health Service Access," *Chinese Health Resources*, no. 6 (2000).

The government should establish medical service standards and technical norms, strengthen the cultivation of professional skills and ethical construction, and improve the service quality and attitude of medical and healthcare staff. It should establish and refine the evaluation system of medical service quality and enhance the supervision and evaluation of public hospitals' medical services by health administrative authorities. At the same time, it should establish an information disclosure system to improve the transparency of the medical service process and accept the supervision of the community and patients.

(5) Rationality of the utilization of medical services. There is a serious shortage and waste of resources. Due to the shortfall in medical investment funds and the absence of a compensation mechanism, most public hospitals still prioritize the pursuit of economic benefits and overemphasize the extended development of hospitals. Some hospitals have induced patients to spend unreasonably on medical treatments through excessive prescriptions and overuse of examinations. As a result, patients' medical costs have remained high.[1]

The government should further increase the price of medical and technical services to reduce hospitals' reliance on income from drugs and examinations. At the same time, medical insurance organizations should play a role in supervising the suppliers and demanders of medical services and eliminating over-consumption. They should effectively control the rapid growth of medical service costs and minimize the unreasonable burden on individuals and the state. For example, a system of rewards and penalties should be set up to monitor the costs of designated medical institutions.

---

1   Zeng Liping, "Conceptualization of Medical Service Prices under Socialist Market Economy," *Chinese Health Resources*, no. 4 (1999).

III. Risk-Sharing Mechanisms for Dangerous Action in Medicine

1. Definition of dangerous action in medicine

Since the seventeenth century, based on the experience of the religious wars, the modern states have been assigned an obligation to protect public life and property within their territories. As a result, the state is bound to remove any danger to the state's internal security, i.e., the obligation of Gefahrenabwehr.[1] This obligation evolved into the state's obligation to legislate against infringement of the fundamental rights of individuals.[2] In other words, the law creates a distinction between security and insecurity. The purpose of the distinction is to identify what is insecure and then remove these insecure factors through the state's intervention.

From this point of view, it is clear that the legal distinction between security and insecurity is built on the primacy of security. Insecurity becomes an object of state intervention, and the state is obliged to legislate to eliminate these insecurities to guarantee security. The intervention must be justified by the everyday rule of thumb that the factors constituting the risk infringe on the legal interest, which means that there is a causal relationship between the two.[3] By means of an explicit rule of causation, the state can determine in advance that certain factors will infringe on legal interests and then take appropriate interventions to prevent the danger from occurring.[4] However, some actions in medical practice are indeed dangerous and cannot be excluded by state-prohibitive legislation. Such actions can be described as dangerous actions in medicine.

Dangerous action in medicine is characterized by the following: (1) Such medical action has the potential to harm legal interests, and that potential

---

1 Udo Di Fabio, *Risikoentscheidunhgen im Rechtsstsaat* (J.C.B. Mohr, 1994), S. 32.
2 Starck, ed., *The Obligation of Protection in Basic Rights: Constitutional Theory and Practice (I)*, tans. Li Jianliang (Taiwan: Xue-Lin Publishing House, 1999).
3 Udo Di Fabio, *Risikoentscheidunhgen im Rechtsstsaat* (J.C.B. Mohr, 1994), S. 85.
4 Ibid., S. 67.

has been demonstrated by existing rules of thumb. Because of this, the legitimacy of the behavior of Gefahrenabwehr can be verified here. (2) Even if a medical practitioner has exercised the duty of due care and has not acted with medical negligence, he or she cannot prevent the actual occurrence of such medical action. (3) Such medical action has the potential to cause harm. However, due to the limitations and dependence of medical means, the state cannot exclude such medical actions from its legislation by virtue of the state's duty to protect.

2. Typical dangerous actions in medicine and their harm to medical justice

Due to the lagging legislation in China, there is no effective risk-sharing mechanism for dangerousness in medicine in the medical industry. The author will only illustrate a few typical types of dangerous medical actions.

> *Experimental action in medicine*

Experimental action in medicine is a special form of medical action, also known as human experimentation. It refers to the conduct of experimental research of medical technology, drugs, or medical devices on human beings for the purpose of developing and improving medical technology and advancing new medical knowledge. Firstly, clinical trials are conducted to find out the effects of the target on the human body, which is a prerequisite for the target to be marketed. The purpose of the direct treatment of the subject becomes secondary. Secondly, clinical trials use targets whose risks and efficacy are unknown. From the results of the trials, we cannot draw logical conclusions from the current medical knowledge acquired by human beings. Thirdly, if a personal injury occurs during a clinical trial, even though the company or medical institution has fulfilled its obligations of adequate notification and prudent monitoring, the company or medical institution will raise the defense that it is not subjectively at fault. Fourthly, even if patients seek judicial remedies as victims, it is rarely feasible to prove the presence of a direct causal relationship between the target and the consequences of the personal injury.

> *Invasive action in medicine*

Many of the drugs, examinations, or surgical procedures that have been used in the past to treat diseases have been found to be not always helpful to the human body as experience and knowledge have been gained. It is accepted by the medical community that medical treatment is inherently invasive to some extent. If the invasive properties exceed the benefits that can be generated from the treatment, the action should be considered invasive in medicine. However, it can hardly be defined by the narrow definition of medical action.

Looking back at the history of clinical trials of human medicines, we can see that some of the new medicines that were used to treat diseases in the past were discovered to be not always beneficial to human beings with the accumulation of relevant medical experience and knowledge. When such medical action is proven to be flawed by the rule of thumb upon its implementation, the recipient of the medical action is entitled to financial compensation. The practitioner may also be able to defend themselves by arguing that they do not commit a subjective medical error when the medical action is performed.

> *Adverse drug reaction*

An adverse drug reaction is a harmful reaction that is unrelated to the purpose of the drug or is unexpected when a qualified drug is used under normal dosage. According to the World Health Organization (WHO), the rate of adverse drug reactions in hospitalized patients ranges from 10% to 20% in various countries, and 5% of these patients die as a result of a severe adverse drug reaction.[1] In the world, about one-third of the deaths of patients are due to improper use of drugs, and deaths caused by adverse drug reactions take up fourth place among the causes of death of the general population. Among the more than 50 million patients hospitalized in China every year, more than 2.5 million are related to adverse drug reactions, and more than 5 million patients have suffered from adverse drug reactions

---

1   Zhuang Shan, "From Chaos to Order in Drug-Related Incidents," *Sanlian Lifeweek*, no. 12 (2002).

during their hospital stay. Adverse drug reactions cause 240,000 deaths per year in China, 11 times the number of deaths caused by the 19 types of major infectious diseases.[1]

According to the statutory concept of adverse drug reaction, the Product Quality Law should not be applied to adverse drug reactions in China's civil law. In other words, the principle of no-fault liability should not be applied to adverse drug reactions. Because an adverse drug reaction is not caused by substandard quality of drugs; on the contrary, the drugs involved in an adverse drug reaction must be qualified and must comply with the national drug standards. What the Product Quality Law regulates is defective drugs. Once an adverse drug reaction case is identified as an "adverse reaction," it has been determined that the drug is in compliance with national drug standards. It thus excludes the application of the Product Quality Law.

> ### *No-fault blood transfusion reaction*

In the process of clinical blood transfusion, as the antigen is produced before the antibody is produced, the hepatitis C virus cannot be detected by the existing technologies and equipment until the antigen has been produced. Still, the antibody has not yet been formed. In the global medical sector, a certain range of omission rates for the Hepatitis C virus is allowed. In China, the permitted omission rate is 3%. Due to the objective factors of the window period and omission rate, it is estimated that absolutely safe blood only accounts for about 40% of the blood transfused. As we can see, no-fault blood transfusion refers to the incident in which the donor, the blood station, and the transfusion provider have all exercised the duty of reasonable care without subjective fault. Still, the recipient is infected due to the limitation of medical technology. In view of the above characteristics, no-fault blood transfusion is not deemed to be among the medical accidents in the Regulation on the Handling of Medical Accidents. In judicial practice, when blood recipients who have been infected file a claim for compensation with the People's Court, in some cases, the claim is dismissed on the grounds that neither the blood station nor the transfusion provider is at fault. In some

---

1   Gao Duo, "When Will the 'Paper Tiger' Stop Acting Aggressively: Concern about Drug-Borne Hazards," *Health Times*, June 6, 2002.

cases, the claim is accommodated through the principle of equity in the General Principles of the Civil Law, whereby the parties concerned have to be jointly liable for the results of the abovementioned damages.

3. Conceptualization of the mechanism of risk sharing

According to the conventional theory of tort law, there are often two principles of attribution of liability for torts: the principle of liability for fault and the principle of no-fault liability. The legal application of the principle of no-fault liability is subject to the legislation of the National People's Congress. However, the principle of liability for dangerous action in medicine mentioned above is not supported by the General Principles of the Civil Law. The principle of liability for fault is often applied, but cases tend to be deadlocked because the party at fault cannot be identified. Currently, most of China's precedents are based on the principle of equity of the General Principles of the Civil Law, whereby the parties concerned share the liability on an equal footing. However, such a way to mediate differences often fails to satisfy the parties concerned. Patients, in particular, do not realize why they are not entitled to financial compensation for their misfortune.

Theoretically, the basic idea of the principle of no-fault liability is not to sanction unlawful behavior, but to reasonably distribute the damages of misfortune. On the basis of a sound and complete insurance system, it aims at socializing the distribution of damages through the insurance system. For this reason, no-fault liability is generally applicable to accidental disasters, such as industrial disasters, traffic accidents, and other cases. These dangerous operations have the following characteristics: (1) They are legal and essential. (2) Accidents happen frequently. (3) They cause huge damage and involve a large number of victims. (4) Most of the accidents are the result of technical defects, which can hardly be prevented. (5) It is difficult for the victims to prove whether the perpetrators have been negligent or not. It can be seen that the above dangerous actions in medicine include experimental medical action, adverse drug reactions, and no-fault blood transfusion. In this regard, it is entirely feasible to establish a new risk-sharing mechanism by means of legislation, with the principle of no-fault liability as the means and the compulsory insurance system in the industry as the guarantee.[1]

IV. Definition of the Act of Spontaneous Agency

The legal relationship in medicine refers to the legal relationship formed when a medical staff member is entrusted by a patient or, for other reasons, performs a medical action such as diagnosis and treatment of the patient. Except for compulsory medical relationships, legal relationships in medicine are civil legal relationships with civil rights and obligations between equal civil subjects, conforming to the requirements of the legal right model stipulated in the civil law. A legal relationship in medicine is usually expressed as a contractual relationship between a patient and a healthcare organization or a healthcare worker. The relationship is established by the free will of the parties, i.e., a medical contract or a contract of diagnosis and treatment.[2] However, there are also legal relationships in medicine that arise from de facto legal acts performed by a medical institution or a medical staff on a patient. According to the provisions of the General Principles of the Civil Law, the spontaneous agency in medical affairs means that medical institutions or medical personnel voluntarily provide medical services to patients in order to prevent damage to the patient's life and health interests in the absence of contractual or legal obligations. It is also commonly known as the act of "Learning from Lei Feng."

However, due to the lack of clarity of health legislation in China, a vast number of medical personnel have a vague and confusing idea of the behavior of spontaneous agency. It directly leads to an inability of medical personnel to foresee the legal consequences of their actions and indirectly constitutes an offense against medical justice. For example, Article 24 of Chapter 3 of the Practice Rules of the Law on Practicing Doctors of the

---

1 Zhu Huai-Zu, *Food and Drugs and Consumer Protection: Doctrines and Case Studies* (Taiwan: Tainan Book Publishing Company, 2000).

2 Li Sheng-Lung, *Introduction to Health Care Laws and Regulations* (Taiwan: Farseeing Publishing Group, 1976).

People's Republic of China (hereinafter referred to as the Law on Practicing Doctors) stipulates that "A physician shall take urgent measures to treat a patient who is in a critical condition; he/she may not refuse to provide emergency treatment." Is it a violation of the Law on Practicing Doctors if a healthcare worker discovers a patient outside the hospital but fails to treat him or her? Should they be held legally liable? If the medical practitioner is a dentist but performs a delivery for a pregnant woman on a train, and the mother and baby die as a result of an error, should the medical practitioner be held legally liable? Do medical personnel have a legal obligation to treat a person who has attempted suicide and is unwilling to seek medical care? Do hospitals have a duty to treat incapacitated patients in "non-urgent cases" directly if no guardian of the patient is present?

Article 24 of the Law on Practicing Doctors is included in Chapter 3 of the Practice Rules. Therefore, the medical staff has every reason to believe that Article 24 only regulates their professional behavior in the hospital. In the author's opinion, it would be appropriate to interpret the above actions pursuant to the provisions of spontaneous agency in the General Principles of the Civil Law. In this way, it can also ease the duty of care of the bona fide administrator in the administration process, and reduce or exempt the damage caused to the administered person by his or her administration actions.[1] A fundamental way to accomplish medical justice is to promulgate the Emergency Care Law of the People's Republic of China as soon as possible and the Mental Health Law of the People's Republic of China and to refine the provisions of the Law on Practicing Doctors.

V. Reservations Regarding the Duty of Explanation or Disclosure

The duties of disclosure and explanation in medicine have become an integral part of the doctor-patient relationship or the payment in the medical contract. The duties of disclosure and explanation in medicine and the pa-

---

1   Wang Zejian, *Principles of the Law of Obligations* (Beijing: China University of Political Science and Law Press, 2001).

tient's informed consent are related to the patient's subjectivity and initiative in medical treatment and the execution of the so-called "human rights in medicine." For this reason, it is particularly imperative to define such duties legally.

Articles 1–2 of Japan's Medical Care Act stipulate that "In providing medical care, a physician, dentist, pharmacist, nurse or other medical care professional must give proper explanations and endeavor to foster understanding in medical care recipients." However, if the patient is suffering from a serious illness such as cancer, should the physician fulfill the duty of disclosure? Since the patient has the right to know about his/her condition, theoretically, the physician is obliged to fulfill his/her duty of explanation and disclosure. However, if the disclosure results in the patient's depression or attempts to commit suicide, should the physician disclose the patient's condition in its entirety? In Japan, the Supreme Court recently ruled on a case in which a physician failed to fulfill the duty of disclosure to a patient and his/her family when the patient was suspected to be suffering from liver cancer. In this regard, the court held that the disclosure of cancer condition concerns the explanation of a specific medical field and is different from the explanation of everyday medical activities, such as the explanation of a common disease such as a cold, the administration of medication, the details of an operation, or the method of nursing care. In principle, physicians should inform patients of their illness, their conditions, the nature and consequences of the medical action, and the possible side effects or dangers involved. That way, the patient will have the ability to make a rational decision. However, if a patient is suffering from an incurable disease or a disease with a low treatment rate, the physician's truthful disclosure of the disease or the result of the cure rate will hit the patient hard and cause him or her to become deeply disturbed, fearful, sad, or self-abandoned, or to commit suicide. When the physician communicates more deeply with the patient, he or she will know the patient better, and the patient will be more cooperative. It will not only enhance the sensitivity of the physician's judgment, but also maximize the use of technologies for the patient and bring out the highest effectiveness of the medical treatment. Such a reservation of an explanation that adversely affects the medical treatment is theoretically referred to as the "therapeutic privilege of the physician."[1] However, the use of therapeutic privilege affects the rights of both physicians and patients. In order to avoid controversy, physicians should, at a minimum, expressly document the use of therapeutic privilege in the medical record as evidence of a failure to fulfill the duties of disclosure and explanation.[2]

Surveys have shown that most medical practitioners and patients' families tend not to inform patients of their illnesses to the fullest extent when patients are critically ill. On the contrary, the same group of individuals, if they are patients, mostly demand to know the truth about the diagnosis, treatment, efficacy, and progression of their diseases.[3] The author imagines that if a patient suffers from stomach cancer, after the operation, his family members discuss with the medical staff to try to keep the real condition unknown to the patient. The patient will definitely end his/her life journey in suspicion, despair, and pain. Medical practitioners tend to give too much consideration to the patient's illness but neglect their social life. The patient may make wrong judgments and choices about his/her job, family, property, and even romance because of the intentional concealment of his/her illness. I believe that the same person, when put in the position of a doctor (or a patient's relative) or a patient, will express opposite opinions about the necessity of concealing their conditions. It also highlights the patient's claim to the right to be informed.

In today's society, where human rights are respected and protected, patients request the right to informed consent, know their own conditions, and make appropriate decisions, which is undoubtedly considered an advancement. In the late 1950s, the US judiciary gradually accepted the principle of "informed consent" and applied it to the patient-physician relationship and clinical practice. Since the 1960s, it has become common practice in both common law and civil law systems to respect the patient's right to informed consent. For example, the US District Court for the District of Kansas held

---

1   Wang Zejian, *Law of Tort* (Beijing: China University of Political Science and Law Press, 2002).

2   Yeung Hui-ling, "Study on the Duty of Explanation of Physicians," Taiwan: The Graduate Institute of Law and Interdisciplinary Studies, National Chengchi University, 1990.

3   Zhu Xiaoli, "A Survey on the Public View of Whether to Inform the Serious Patients of Their Real Conditions," *Medicine and Philosophy*, no. 8 (2005).

that a physician has a duty to reasonably inform a patient of the nature and results of the treatment that has been revealed or recommended, as well as to disclose dangerous conditions that may be associated with the treatment as understood by the physician.[1] A survey of 2,500 patients was conducted in an outpatient clinic at the University of Kansas Medical Center. It was concluded that most patients wanted their physicians to inform them of all the adverse effects of their medications and did not agree that their physicians had reservations about these effects.[2]

The patient's informed consent and the physician's disclosure of information in medical service activities have become the rights and obligations conferred by the law. However, Article 26 of the Law on Practicing Doctors stipulates that a physician shall truthfully inform the patient or his/her family members of the patient's condition, but shall take care to avoid unfavorable consequences for the patient. In Article 11 of the Regulation on the Handling of Medical Accidents, it is also provided that in the course of medical activities, medical institutions, and their medical staff shall truthfully inform patients of their medical conditions, medical treatments, and the risks of medical treatment, and shall answer their inquiries promptly; however, they shall avoid any unfavorable consequences to the patients. Unlike in Europe and the United States, Chinese society still recognizes and accepts such reservations about the right to be informed. In the author's opinion, it cannot be denied that they have misunderstood and distorted medical justice. As early as 1993, the WHO proposed the following strategies for doctors to inform: (1) Doctors should have a plan in advance. (2) They should leave room for maneuver when informing patients of their illnesses so that patients can have a chance to accept their conditions step by step. (3) They should inform the patient in several sessions. (4) They should give the patient as much hope as possible when informing them of their illnesses. (5) They should not deceive the patient. (6) During the notification process,

---

1   Duan Kuang and He Xiangyu, "Doctors' Duty to Inform and Patients' Commitment. Liang Huixing," in *Collection of Essays on Civil and Commercial Law*, vol. 12 (Beijing: Law Press China, 1999).

2   Zieglerdk, "How Much Information about the Side Effect of Medicine Should the Doctors Inform the Patients," *Archintern Med* (2001): 161.

they should allow the patient to fully ventilate their emotions, and treat them promptly. (7) After the notification of the disease, they should work together with the patient to develop a plan for their future life and treatment and maintain close and further contact with the patient. For cancer patients, when they have become highly suspicious of their malignant tumors, but cannot be convinced, they will be even more anxious or worried than those who have already been informed of their cancer.[1] In the author's opinion, it is a general trend to inform patients of their conditions and protect their right to informed consent in terms of law, reason, and sentiment. Physicians should not only truthfully inform critically ill patients of their conditions, but also overcome resistance and shorten the time it takes for society to recognize the fulfillment of the right of physicians to inform and the right of patients to give informed consent.

It must be recognized that medical relationships are complicated, and the problems they generate are likely to be specific from one to another. There may not be a coherent or subordinate relationship between them. As a result, when it comes to the individual problems of medical justice, it seems that the specific connotation of justice in medical cases has yet to be explored as to how to make value trade-offs.

---

1   Montgomery C. et al., "Psychological Distress among Cancer Patients and Informed Consent," *Psychosom Res* 46, no. 3 (1999): 241–245.

On Hospital Service Contracts

For a long time, doctors have been practicing medicine in order to help patients as if they were their own family members. The patients often return
the favor by considering the doctors as present-day Hua Tuo and having a
benevolent mind and heart. The relationship between the doctors and the
patients can be described as cordial. However, with the development of the
market economy, the ethical relationship between doctors and patients has
become increasingly indifferent. In some cases, doctors and patients have
even turned against each other and ended up in court. A balance has to be
found between rescuing the world and fulfilling the legal obligations. They
must re-conceptualize many basic concepts of legal relationships in medicine and carry out supporting legislative reforms. In the author's opinion,
while discussing the various manifestations of medical disputes, it is necessary to analyze the basic concepts, such as hospital service contracts, and
explore the legal theoretical basis for resolving various medical disputes.

I. Legal Relationships in Medicine

1. The concept of legal relationships in medicine

Legal relationships in medicine refer to the legal relationships formed by
medical workers who are entrusted by patients or for other reasons to perform medical acts such as diagnosis and treatment of patients. Except for
compulsory medical relationships, legal relationships in medicine are civil
legal relationships with civil rights and obligations formed between equal

civil subjects and meet the requirements of the legal model stipulated in the civil law. Legal relationships in medicine result from adjusting the personal and property relationships between doctors and patients in accordance with the civil law accompanying medical acts. At the same time, it is a product of the combination of personal and property relations between doctors and patients and the forms of civil law.

2. Types of legal relationships in medicine

According to the requirements for the establishment of legal relationships in medicine, the rights and obligations of the parties involved, and the corresponding legal liabilities, legal relationships in medicine can be further subdivided into the following three categories:

> *Relationships in hospital service contracts*

Legal relationships in medicine are usually expressed as contractual relationships between patients and medical institutions or individual medical practitioners. These relationships are formed through the free will of the parties, i.e., hospital service contracts or medical contracts. Hospital service contracts are established like contracts in general after an offer is made and consent is given. In other words, a hospital service contract is concluded when a patient makes an offer of medical treatment, and a medical practitioner accepts the offer as a commitment.

> *Spontaneous agency relationship*

However, there are also legal relationships arising from de facto medical and legal acts of a medical institution or an individual medical practitioner towards a patient. This situation constitutes a spontaneous agency relationship between the medical institution or the individual medical practitioner and the patient. Article 93 of the General Principles of the Civil Law of the People's Republic of China provides that "If a person acts as manager or provides services in order to protect another person's interests when he is not legally or contractually obligated to do so, he shall be entitled to claim from the beneficiary the expenses necessary for such assistance." Spontaneous agency is the act of serving as a manager when a person is not legally or contractually obligated to do so. Spontaneous agency in medical affairs is the act of a medical institution or a medical staff member voluntarily providing medical services for a patient in order to prevent the patient's life and health interests from being jeopardized, when they are not legally or contractually obligated to do so. The spontaneous agency relationship in medical affairs is common in three circumstances: (1) Medical personnel discover a patient outside the hospital and treat him or her. (2) A hospital or medical personnel treats a person who is unwilling to seek medical attention after a suicide attempt. (3) In the absence of a guardian, a hospital or a medical staff member directly provides diagnosis and treatment to a patient with no or limited capacity to act and who is "not in acute danger."

> *Compulsory relationships in medicine*

The most special of the legal relationships in medicine is that the state, based on the special nature of medical treatment and the protection of people's lives and physical health, legally confers on medical institutions the obligation to provide compulsory treatment and on patients to receive compulsory treatment. It is an authorized exercise of public power, and the medical institution is only a client, an agent of the state. Legal relationships in medicine are present between the state and the patient, and such legal relationships in medicine can be referred to as compulsory relationships in medicine.

II. Nature of Hospital Service Contracts

Hospital service contracts are contracts with the content of medical treatment. Although medical treatment requires health and medical workers to acquire special skills, knowledge, or technology, it is also based on specific acts as its content. For this reason, hospital service contracts are essentially considered to be labor contracts. According to the general theory, labor contracts are classified into three types depending on the purpose of payment for labor, the presence or absence of remuneration, or the independent performance of labor by the labor supplier: employment contracts, work contracts, and commission contracts. There is no consensus among countries as to which type of labor contract a hospital service contract belongs to.

1. The doctrine of quasi-commission contracts

The doctrine is generally recognized in Japanese doctrine and jurisprudence. According to this doctrine, a hospital service contract is a contract
that provides appropriate medical treatment after the cause or term of the
patient's disease is quickly and accurately diagnosed by utilizing the physician's knowledge and skill in clinical medicine. As long as there is no special
agreement, the achievement of a good result cannot be included in the content of the obligations. According to the Civil Code of Japan, commission
contracts are limited to legal acts, while medical treatment is essentially a
factual act, not a legal act. For this reason, this type of contract can only
be called a quasi-commission contract. Hospital service contracts are completely different from contracts with resultant obligations, which aim to pay
objects and whose contents are determined to achieve a specific result. A
hospital service contract is an "obligation of means" to treat an injury or
disease with the contents of giving prudent care and practicing appropriate
diagnostic and therapeutic actions. In other words, the patient entrusts the
medical staff to handle the diagnostic and therapeutic affairs of the disease,
and the physician especially handles them, thus entering into a quasi-commission contract.

2. The doctrine of commission contracts

This is the general statement of the legal and practical communities in
Taiwan, China. It holds that the civil law of Taiwan does not distinguish between legal acts and de facto acts in relation to commission contracts. A
commission contract can be entered into irrespective of whether the matter
being dealt with is a legal or non-legal act. As a result, it is argued that hospital service contracts should be regarded as commission contracts in general.
Only when the patient and the physician agree to pay for the cure of the
disease is the contract treated as a contract for work.

3. The doctrine of work contracts

According to this doctrine, although hospital service contracts are not for
the cure of diseases (the general case without special agreement), the physi-

cian is obliged to complete the medical treatment. Such "completion" of the medical treatment is the purpose of hospital service contracts. As such, "resultant obligations" refers to the completion of the medical treatment itself, regardless of whether the disease is cured or not. Work contracts emphasize that payment is made only when some tasks are accomplished. Therefore, a hospital service contract is a contract for work if it is agreed that the completion of a certain operation or the cure of a specific disease is the basis for payment. In Japanese practice, it has been ruled that surgical treatment of duodenal ulcers is "a contract for work to perform ulcer operations." It should be noted that the contract for work in this case is not the same as the contract for work where there is a special agreement to "cure a disease."

4. The doctrine of employment contracts

It is a general statement in Germany. In the Civil Code of Germany, commission contracts are limited to gratuitous acts, whereas hospital service contracts are usually characterized by gratuitous acts. Therefore, hospital service contracts cannot be interpreted as commission contracts. Consequently, these contracts can only be interpreted as employment contracts for the labor of others. In some countries in the common law system, hospital service contracts are also commonly interpreted as employment contracts.

5. The doctrine of anonymous service contracts

It is argued that the categorization of hospital service contracts into contracts for work and quasi-commission contracts fails to encompass all hospital service contracts. It seems appropriate to regard hospital service contracts as quasi-commission contracts from the perspective of the purpose of the patient's entrustment to the physician for the proper performance of the diagnostic and therapeutic services. However, if we analyze the characteristics of hospital service contracts, we may find that there is a big difference between hospital service contracts and typical commission contracts, so it is hard to define hospital service contracts as a typical commission contract. It is more reasonable to call it an anonymous service contract.

Combined with the actual situation in China, the author carefully analyzes the above doctrines and considers that all of them are defective. As for the doctrine of quasi-commission contracts, China's laws have not made the distinction and limitation between legal acts and factual acts on commission contracts. Commission contracts can be established regardless of whether the affairs dealt with are legal acts or non-legal acts. Therefore, there is no basis for establishing a quasi-commission contract. Similarly, in China's civil law, commission services can be either paid or unpaid. For this reason, it is inappropriate to apply the employment contract doctrine of Germany, Britain, and the United States. A detailed analysis of the commission contract suggests that it is not entirely consistent with the provisions of the contract law in China. First of all, the principal should pay the cost of the commissioned affairs in advance. However, hospital service contracts are not purely property contracts, so physicians cannot defend against simultaneous fulfillment before the patient pays for them. Secondly, the agent should handle the commissioned affairs according to the principal's instructions. However, hospital service contracts are characterized by their professionalism, and the patients cannot instruct the medical staff on how to administer the medical treatment. Thirdly, the agent should report on handling the commissioned affairs as requested by the principal. In medical practice, physicians tend to deliberately conceal the true condition of a patient who is terminally ill. With regard to the doctrine of work contracts, it cannot be applied to general hospital service contracts that do not emphasize the effectiveness of medical treatment, except for the case where it is agreed that the payment will be made only when a specific operation is completed or the patient is cured, which is in line with the characteristics of the doctrine of work contracts.

To sum up, all of the above doctrines are defective, and the author believes that it is hard to cover hospital service contracts with any single type of contract in the law of obligations, given the specificity and professionalism of medical treatment and the fact that medical personnel are also subject to the regulation of medical ethics. In countries where medicine and pharmaceuticals are not separated from each other, hospital service contracts should be defined according to their contents and should not be generalized:

(1) A contract for payment of remuneration for the completion of a specific operation or cure of an illness is a paid contract in which the payment of remuneration is conditional on the completion of a specific task. In addition, the medical staff decides the method

of operation based on his/her independent judgment. In this case, hospital service contracts fully meet the requirements of work contracts and should be recognized as contracts for work.

(2) With regard to hospital service contracts in general outpatient clinics, China has not yet adopted the system of separation of medicine and pharmaceuticals, and medical institutions, in addition to the provision of diagnosis or treatment, sell prescription drugs at the same time. Thus, the hospital service contracts in general outpatient clinics should be a mixture of anonymous service contracts and sales contracts.

(3) Hospital service contracts for hospitalization are extremely complex, involving the provision of consultation and treatment services, the rental of wards and equipment, the supply of medicines, equipment, blood, and meals, and the employment of caregivers. Therefore, hospital service contracts for hospitalization should be a mixture of anonymous service contracts, lease contracts, sale contracts, and employment contracts.

(4) Patients receive experimental medical treatment, and on the one hand, medical institutions offer experimental medical services. On the other hand, the patient receives medical services free of charge or receives an organ donation. Hospital service contracts are a mixture of anonymous service contracts and gift contracts.

(5) A health checkup is intended only for judging health conditions and detecting diseases, but not for diagnosing or treating diseases, so it is a simple labor service for a health checkup provided by a medical service provider. For this reason, such hospital service contracts are anonymous service contracts.

III. Categories and Characteristics of Hospital Service Contracts

1. Categories of hospital service contracts

Hospital service contracts can be categorized into four types depending on the purpose and content of the diagnosis and treatment.

> *General hospital service contracts*

Contracts for the purpose of diagnosis and treatment of diseases, with payments made for outpatient, hospitalization, and surgical treatment services.

> *Contracts for health checks*

Contracts for the purpose of early detection of disease or knowledge of the health condition, whereby it is agreed to have a health checkup performed by a healthcare service provider.

> *Experimental hospital service contracts*

These contracts can be divided into two types: experimental acts for diagnostic and therapeutic purposes and acts for purely experimental purposes. The former is basically the same as general medical treatment, but the means utilized is a newly invented diagnostic or therapeutic method or drug, or the effect is not fully determined in medicine, or it is covered by the general concept of diagnosis and treatment. The latter refers to human experimentation, and such contracts, although related to advances in medicine, have nothing to do with diagnosis and treatment.

> *Special hospital service contracts*

They are contracts in which the person who needs medical services does not have a health problem and receives services from a medical service provider. With the development of medical technology, the scope of development of many medical fields has greatly exceeded the purpose of diagnosis and treatment. For example, there are plastic surgeries solely for cosmetic purposes, transsexual operations, and abortions for non-therapeutic purposes. These behaviors are not for medical purposes, but even for destructive purposes.

Euthanasia, on the other hand, is even closer to the core of medical ethics, challenging the professional morality that physicians "must not jeopardize the health of human beings with what they have learned."

Regardless of the categorization of hospital service contracts, it does not affect the rights and obligations arising from them. There is only a slight difference in that the chance of medical accidents may be lower (contracts for health checks), and the duty of care may be heavier (experimental hospital service contracts).

2. Characteristics of hospital service contracts

Hospital service contracts differ from other types of contracts in terms of the content of the payment and the person to whom the payment is made. The content of the payment is characterized by the invasive, life-saving, and specialized properties of the medical treatment that is subject to the payment. The object of payment is characterized by the direct connection between the diagnostic and therapeutic act and the body and the absence of a guarantee of the medical result due to the objective reasons for the impossibility of domination. Thus, hospital service contracts are characterized as follows.

> *Exclusivity of hospital service contracts on the qualification of contracting subjects*

In a market economy, the qualifications of subjects of contracts are relatively loosened, and the government hardly imposes any restrictions. However, due to the nature of medical treatment, which requires special knowledge, it is strictly exclusive. The exclusivity is manifested in the use of the name of the physician and the practice of medicine. The use of the term "physician" implies that an individual may only refer to themselves as a physician or specialist physician if they are certified and licensed as a medical practitioner (including nurse practitioners). The practice of medicine means that a person is prohibited from practicing medicine if he/she is not qualified as a medical practitioner (nurse). Since medical treatment is related to the health and lives of patients and cannot be performed by those who do not have specialized medical knowledge, the licensing system is designed to exclude those who have not received sufficient education and training from practicing medicine.

> **Restrictions on the autonomy of will in hospital service contracts under public law**

The autonomy of will is a fundamental principle of civil law. The parties have the right to choose the counterparty, to decide the content of the contract, and to modify or amend the contract when concluding a contract, and are not subject to the interference of public law. Hospital service contracts are contracts under private law, and the parties should be entitled to these freedoms of will. However, due to the moral nature of medical treatment, the autonomy of the will of the parties, especially the medical practitioner, is subject to the constraints of public law. The Medical Law of Japan stipulates that a physician cannot refuse a patient's request for diagnosis and treatment without a justifiable reason. Even if the disease for which the patient is requesting treatment is outside of the physician's area of specialization, the physician cannot refuse. The provision of "compulsory contractual obligation" in public law is based on the social responsibility of physicians to treat the sick and to save people. It is intended to fully protect the patient's right to life and health. In addition, there are restrictions on the medical practitioner in deciding and altering the contract's content.

> **Legality and morality in hospital service contracts**

Medical treatment involves healing the wounded, rescuing the dying, and curing the sickness to save the patient. Medical treatment of physicians must be regulated by medical morality or medical ethics. Medical ethics has a very long history, with the most famous being the Hippocratic Oath, "I will prescribe regimen for the good of my patients according to my ability and my judgment and never do harm to anyone." It is the oath that every medical student must take upon graduation. With the development of medicine, the norms of medical treatment have been enriched and improved by the medical profession. The Declaration of Geneva, adopted by the World Medical Association in 1948, requires physicians to "practice medicine out of conscience and with dignity" and to "care most for the health of their patients." The Declaration of Helsinki of 1964 also states that "the protection of the health of the people" is the mission of physicians.

Medical ethics, as a self-regulatory mechanism for actors and a system of societal evaluation, has been widely elevated to laws. The ethical norms of physicians have become their duties, such as the duty of diagnosis and treatment, the duty of referral, and the duty of explanation. In addition, the introduction of new medical technologies and concepts has led to new problems in the field of medical ethics, such as perinatal genetics, in vitro fertilization, brain death, euthanasia, organ transplantation, and AIDS. These problems have aroused great concern and reflection among the public and the legislators.

> *The specialization of medical obligations and the inequality between the parties concerned*

Diagnosis and treatment, as elements of payments in hospital service contracts, require physicians to acquire a high degree of specialized knowledge and skills. This characteristic determines the inequality of capacity between the two parties to a hospital service contract. While the physician, a party to the contract, is a medical expert, the patient, as the other party to the contract, is usually an ordinary person with no medical knowledge. It implies that the patient, who is a party to the contract, cannot agree on the details of the diagnosis and treatment because he or she is not aware of the obligation of the physician based on the contract, i.e., the diagnosis and treatment. In this case, the patient can only expect the physician to administer a diagnosis and treatment that is deemed medically appropriate by the physician out of conscience and morals.

> *Abstract and instrumental aspects of medical obligations*

The contractual obligation of the physician is the medical treatment itself, and the abstract nature of the medical obligation is expressed in the phrase "to administer medically appropriate diagnosis and treatment." In order to evaluate whether the diagnosis and treatment are appropriate, it is necessary to examine and evaluate the whole process of diagnosis and treatment, not only each diagnosis and treatment action. Because of the complexity of human tissue function and the unpredictability of the patient, the diagnosis and treatment acts are uncertain. For this reason, each and every specific diagnostic and therapeutic act performed during the whole process of diagnosis and treatment cannot be specified from the beginning. The physician can only choose and perform the appropriate medical act based on the actual situation at a certain time and in a certain context.

The instrumental nature of medical obligations refers to the fact that both the whole process of medical treatment and each specific act of diagnosis and treatment are rarely "obligations of result" to achieve a specific result, but can only be used to treat a disease. This is due to the uncertainty of the act of diagnosis and treatment, and it is also because not all diseases can be conquered by modern medicine.

> ### Collaboration between the parties

The performance of any contract requires the collaboration of both parties. However, the collaboration of the parties is particularly important in the case of a medical contract, because the diagnosis and treatment is carried out by the patient, who is a party to the contract. The patient's collaboration is essential to the proper administration of the diagnosis and treatment. For example, the patient is required to answer questions correctly and in detail when asked by the physician, and the patient is required to follow the physician's instructions regarding medication and maintenance.

> ### Physicians' respect for patients' right to make decisions

Because of the highly specialized nature of medical treatment, physicians have a high degree of discretion in their practice. They do not have to follow the patients' requests and instructions to fulfill their obligations. Since diagnosis and treatment are carried out on the patient's own life and body, which are irreplaceable and usually cause physical intrusion and pain to the patient, the two parties are unable to agree on the outcome of the medical treatment. With the advancement of social culture and civilization and the popularization of medical knowledge, more and more patients request to participate in their medical treatment. For this reason, respecting patients' autonomy has become an important principle of medical ethics and the basis for building a modern doctor-patient relationship. The patient has the "right to be informed" by the medical practitioner about the cause of his/her illness, the methods of diagnosis, the principles of treatment, and the possible prognosis of his/her illness. Furthermore, the patient has the "right" to agree or disagree with the physician's treatment decisions. In this context, the physician is obliged to respect the patient's autonomy. Hence, the theory of informed consent has been introduced.

IV. Establishment and Entry into Force of Hospital Service Contracts

The Contract Law of the People's Republic of China provides that a contract is established when the parties express their mutual agreement on their intentions, regardless of whether it is express or implied. The so-called mutual agreement of intention refers to the agreement of parties in opposition, that is, the agreement of the offer and the acceptance. The two opposing parties only need to agree on the necessary points to establish the contract; the contract can be presumed to be established even if the non-essential points have not been indicated.

Notice Obligation of Hospital and Doctor as Spontaneous Agency

[CASE] September 25, 2001, Person A, a villager from Shaanxi Province who was doing business alone in Guangzhou, did not pay for the cab, and the driver asked the police to help him collect the money. Seeing Person A's abnormal mental condition, the police sent him to Guangzhou Municipal Psychiatric Hospital, where he was diagnosed with "schizophrenia." Person A was then transferred to the Guangzhou Baiyun Psychiatric Rehabilitation Hospital, which temporarily admitted unemployed migrant people with diseases. After being hospitalized, Person A refused to take any food. In addition to symptomatic treatment and nursing care, the medical staff used nasal feeding to implement the supporting treatment, but every time, it was strongly resisted by Person A. Whenever the medical staff asked him to take a meal, Person A made a lot of noise and shouted all day long, getting into fights with patients in the same ward. Half a month later, Person A suffered from frequent diarrhea and red jelly-like stools. The doctor suspected that Person A was suffering from an "organic mental disorder combined with toxic dysentery." To prevent Person A's intracranial pressure from increasing, the doctors started to control the amount of infusion he was given. However, his condition deteriorated, and he died 17 days later.

Person A's body was autopsied by the Forensic Medical Identification Center of Sun Yat-sen University, and the conclusion was that he died of starvation. At the same time, a fist-sized mass of grayish-white tumor was found inside the skull, which had severely compressed his brain tissue. Based on the results of the autopsy, the family members of the deceased sued Baiyun Psychiatric Rehabilitation Hospital on the grounds of "serious negligence in diagnosis, treatment and care of the patient." Also, they claimed for various damages. The Baiyun District Court of Guangzhou held that during Person A's hospitalization, he was in a state of starvation because he refused to eat. At the same time, the hospital failed to take proper medical measures, such as the timely injection of dextrose. As a result, Person A died of starvation. The hospital also failed to take timely action in the fight between Person A and a patient in the same ward, causing Person A to be injured several times and accelerating his death. Therefore, the hospital was grossly negligent. On April 30, 2003, the Baiyun District Court ruled that the Baiyun Psychiatric Rehabilitation Hospital should compensate Person A's family for damages amounting to about RMB 100,000.[1]

I. Legal Relationship between the Patient and the Hospital

"The law is the rule of rights and obligations." So before we discuss a case, we must figure out the legal relationship between the parties, because the parties are entitled to different rights and have different obligations depending on the legal relationship.

In fact, the treatment and management of some patients with mental illness, infectious diseases, and alcoholism should have been harmonized into the category of "compulsory treatment by the state." It is because, unlike other ordinary patients, the illness or abnormal state of these special groups of patients is hazardous to individuals and affects the public interest. Therefore, the state is obliged to limit the private rights of such special groups of people through public power by means of lawful legislative procedures. For example, the Law of the People's Republic of China on Prevention and Treatment of Infectious Diseases stipulates that "When medical care and health institutions and anti-epidemic agencies find infectious diseases, they shall promptly take the following control measures: Patients and pathogen carriers of A Class infectious diseases and patients of AIDS and pulmonary

---

1   Anonymous, "What Is the Responsibility of Hospitals," *Health Daily*, no. 6 (April 27, 2004).

anthrax as a type of anthrax among B Class infectious diseases shall be isolated for treatment. The period of isolation shall be determined according to the medical examination results. For those who refuse treatment in isolation or break away from treatment in isolation before the expiration of the isolation period, the public security department may assist medical care institutions in taking measures to enforce the treatment in isolation." However, to date, China has not yet enacted any legislation on mental health by the National People's Congress, which has caused a lot of inconvenience in practice. It is also hard to define what kind of legal relationship should be between doctors and patients. In view of the current state of mental health legislation in China, the author believes that the relationship between Person A and Guangzhou Baiyun Psychiatric Rehabilitation Hospital should be a spontaneous agency relationship.

Generally speaking, a legal relationship in medicine is a contractual relationship between patients and medical institutions or medical personnel. However, there are also legal relationships arising from de facto medical and legal acts of a medical institution or medical personnel towards a patient. This situation constitutes a spontaneous agency relationship between the medical institution or medical staff and the patient. Article 93 of the General Principles of the Civil Law of the People's Republic of China provides that "If a person acts as manager or provides services in order to protect another person's interests when he is not legally or contractually obligated to do so, he shall be entitled to claim from the beneficiary the expenses necessary for such assistance." The act of serving as a manager when a person is not legally or contractually obligated to do so is a spontaneous agency, commonly known as the act of learning from Lei Feng. Spontaneous agency in medical affairs is the act of a medical institution or a medical staff member voluntarily providing medical services for a patient in order to prevent the patient's life and health interests from being jeopardized when they are not legally or contractually obligated to do so. As a result, the act of management generates a debtor-creditor relationship between the physician and the patient. The spontaneous agency relationship in medical affairs is common in three circumstances: (1) Medical personnel discover a patient outside the hospital and treat him or her. (2) A hospital or medical personnel treats a person who is unwilling to seek medical attention after a suicide attempt. (3) In the absence of a guardian, a hospital or a medical staff member directly provides diagnosis and treatment to a patient with no or limited capacity to act and who is "not in acute danger."[1]

In this case, Baiyun Psychiatric Rehabilitation Hospital, which is a private hospital, did not have a contractual obligation to continue providing medical services for Person A after he was released from the "acute" symptoms. So, is there a contractual obligation between the doctor and the patient? Person A is a patient with mental illness who has no or limited civil capacity and cannot be regarded as the subject of a hospital service contract. The subject of a hospital service contract can only be the guardian of Person A. That is why Person A is called the recipient of medical service, and his guardian is called the demander of medical service in Japan and Taiwan, China. So, how do we look at the act of sending Person A to the hospital by the relevant administrative department? In the author's opinion, such an act should not be an administrative act according to the existing legal system in China. As we all know, administrative acts should have a clear legal basis, as it is said that "the government shall not act without express authorization from the law." As a result, the administrative department's act of sending Person A to the hospital cannot be regarded as an administrative act. To sum up, it can be seen that the hospital should be recognized as a spontaneous agency for providing medical services to avoid harming Person A's life and health interests in the absence of statutory and contractual obligations.

Some people recognize the nature of this case as an act of rescue, and the author believes that this is not appropriate. The act of rescue and justifiable defense are the two systems established by China's criminal law to eliminate unlawful acts. According to Article 21(1) of the Criminal Law of the People's Republic of China, an act of rescue is not to be borne for damage resulting from an act of urgent danger prevention that must be undertaken in order to avert the occurrence of present danger to the state or public interest or the rights of the person, property rights, or other rights of the actor or other people, which impairs the lawful rights and interests of a third party. The object of the act of rescue can only be the legitimate interests of a third party, meaning that the public interest and the legitimate interests of

1 Li Shenglong, *Introduction to Healthcare Regulations* (Taiwan: Farseeing Publishing Group, 1976), 33–36.

oneself or others are preserved by compromising the legitimate interests of an innocent person. It is evident that, during medical treatment, the hospital seldom jeopardizes the legal rights of another minor party. For this reason, it is not appropriate to interpret the rights and obligations under the civil legal relationship in this case by using the act of rescue system of the criminal law.

II. Duty of Care for Hospitals as Managers in Spontaneous Agency Relationships

The managers of spontaneous agency have no obligation to manage their own affairs, but once the managers do so, they should manage them well. It is an inevitable requirement of the law to protect the lawful interests of civil subjects and to maintain the social and economic order. It is also an inevitable result of the fact that the spontaneous agency has become a lawful act. The medical institutions in the legal relationship of the spontaneous agency should uphold the duty of care in good faith. That is to say, medical institutions and medical practitioners should show a high degree of bona fide to the life and health interests of the managed person in the process of medical service and respect the person's personality interests.[1] Specifically, the author holds that the duty of care should cover the following aspects.

1. The duty of adequate management

This duty is manifested in three aspects: (1) The manager should not manage against his or her own will and should manage pursuant to a presumption of his or her own will. In other words, depending on the circumstances of the case, he or she should not manage contrary to what he or she can be presumed to know. It is obvious that the act of treating Person A can be presumed to be the intention of his guardian, so it is clear that the hospital's act of treating him is not contrary to his own intention. (2) The manager should manage Person A in a way that is favorable to him/her. As a result, the way

---

1   Shi Shangkuan, *General Introduction to Debt Law* (Beijing: China University of Political Science and Law Press, 2000), 57–66.

the hospital manages Person A should be in favor of Person A. However, in this case, the hospital was clearly at fault in its rescue behavior. Also, whether the hospital's management is in Person A's interest should be determined by whether it can objectively prevent Person A's interests from being jeopardized. If the hospital subjectively believes that its management method is in the interest of Person A, its management cannot be deemed appropriate. (3) Management should be continued as required by the person's interests. That is to say, if the hospital stops or passively manages Person A to the detriment of his interests, the hospital has the obligation to continue to manage and must not stop managing. Apparently, the hospital, in this case, is also at fault in this respect.[1]

2. Duty of the manager to notify the person concerned of the fact of management

The manager should notify the client of the commencement of the management after the commencement of the management. If the manager does not know who the client is, does not know the client's address, or is unable to notify him/her for other reasons, he/she is not obliged to notify him/her. If waiting for the client's instructions would jeopardize the client's interests, the manager should not wait for the instructions but should manage the case directly. The hospital should also be obliged to notify the guardian of Person A of the fact of management after Person A arrives at the hospital.[2]

3. Duty to compensate for losses caused by improper management by the manager

Article 93 of the General Principles of the Civil Law of the People's Republic of China does not stipulate the compensation obligation of the manager for spontaneous agency, and some people do not think that the manager

---

1   Wang Zejian, *Principles of Debt Law* (Beijing: China University of Political Science and Law Press, 2001), 339–348.

2   Jiang Ping, *Civil Law* (Beijing: China University of Political Science and Law Press, 2000), 721–723.

has such an obligation. According to the author, the manager's obligation to compensate should be generated pursuant to the failure to fulfill other obligations as stated in Article 106(1) of the Law, which states that "citizens and legal persons who breach a contract or fail to fulfill other obligations shall bear civil liability." The principle of liability for fault should apply when determining the duty of compensation. Managers should be liable for compensation only for damage caused by the faulty conduct of their own management. The fault of the manager should be determined on the basis of whether the manager has fulfilled his or her duty of care in managing the affairs. The standard of the manager's duty of care should be subject to the care of a "bona fide manager."

Therefore, if the hospital causes harm to Person A due to deliberate intent or gross negligence (which should be limited to liability negligence) during the course of spontaneous agency, it indicates that the nature of the spontaneous agency behavior has changed. That is, the act of spontaneous agency has been transformed into an act of tort, and the hospital no longer provides medical services for the benefit of Person A, but wrongfully infringes upon Person A's rights and interests. As a result, the hospital should be held liable for tort. But how could it be determined that the hospital's spontaneous agency behavior has been transformed into a tort? In the author's view, the key is to judge the hospital's degree of care and fault. On the one hand, the spontaneous agency behavior is an act encouraged by the law. From the perspective of encouraging such behavior, it should not require too much of a degree of care for that hospital to engage in managerial activities. In general, a hospital should be deemed to have fulfilled its duty of care as long as it handles its affairs in accordance with the duty of care required of a "bona fide manager." In a state of urgency where there is no time for delay, the hospital should not be deemed to have committed a tort as long as it does not act with malice or without regard to the patient's interests, even if it commits ordinary negligence. On the other hand, because the content of the duty of care in civil law is often affected by the relationship of interest, hospitals do not seek benefits for themselves when they engage in management activities, but act in the interest of Person A. For this reason, the requirements for the hospital's duty of care should not be too high. That is to say, if Person A is in a very urgent situation, the medical behavior of the hospital should not be deemed as a tort as long as it is not grossly negligent, even if it causes damage. However, in this case, if the facts are true that "Person A's physical condition deteriorated and he died 17 days later" and that "the hospital failed to take timely measures against Person A's fights with patients in the same ward, causing him to be injured several times," it can hardly be concluded that the hospital had fulfilled its duty as a "bona fide manager." Thus, the author considers that the judgment made by the Baiyun District Court is no fault.

At the same time, this case also reflects the problem of lagging health legislation in China from another aspect. The United States, Japan, and other countries have specialized mental health laws that specify the compulsory identification of some patients with mental illness, the system of hospitalization and treatment, as well as the requirements for hospitals to treat patients with mental illness. For example, it provides that when the police find or receive a report to the police, the police shall immediately escort a person with a mental illness or suspected mental illness to a mental health institution designated by the health authorities for medical treatment if the person is found to cause obvious harm to others or himself or if the person has committed an act of harm. Also, the police shall immediately notify the competent local department of health. If the identity of the person suffering from mental illness or suspected to be suffering from mental illness is ascertained, his/her guardian or family member shall be notified immediately. If the patient or his/her family members are financially disadvantaged and cannot afford the medical expenses, the governments at all levels should make budgetary provisions to subsidize, at their discretion, the medical expenses of patients with serious illnesses during their hospitalization and compulsory hospitalization. These expenses shall be borne by the central government. It is reported that the Mental Health Law of the People's Republic of China has been included in the recent legislative program. It is hoped that the law will be enacted as soon as possible.

Legislation to Promote Hospital Management Mode and Medical Service Mode Transformation

Prompt revision to conflicts between the Regulations on Medical Accident Treatment and the Tort Liability Law was called. The State Council has officially launched the revision of the Regulations on Medical Accidents, the new law tentatively titled the Medical Dispute Prevention and Handling Regulations, a name that suggests the focus of the legislation. The Legislative Affairs Office of the State Council of the People's Republic of China has solicited opinions nationwide on the Medical Dispute Prevention and Handling Regulations (Draft for Review) through the Chinese Government's Legislative Information Network (http://www.chinalaw.gov.cn).

I. Necessity of Amending the Regulations on Medical Accident Treatment

1. Objective need after the Tort Liability Law

The Tort Liability Law was reviewed and passed by the Standing Committee of the National People's Congress on December 26, 2009, and came into effect on July 1, 2010. Elven provisions in Chapter VII on medical damage liability have stipulated relief rules for medical damage liability, fundamentally reformed the dual system of medical damage relief consisting of three dual-track systems: "medical malpractice liability" and "medical negligence liability," and outputted a unified medical injury relief system,[1] quite different from the Regulations on Medical Accident Treatment and supporting clauses applied to handling medical disputes in the past. As the Tort Liability Law landed, the Regulations on Medical Accident Treatment ceased to be the main basis for people's courts to adjudicate medical disputes and civil cases. Still, it reassumed its main legal function as administrative regulations, that is, as the legal basis for the competent health administration department to handle medical accident disputes and investigate administrative responsibilities of administrative management counterparties (medical institutions and medical personnel). From this, it was essential to upgrade the Regulations on Medical Accident Treatment and delete its civil compensation and inconsistency against the Tort Liability Law.

2. Objective need for a two-track system for the evaluation of medical dispute cases

The Regulations on Medical Accident Treatment implemented in 2002 set a medical malpractice technical assessment system under the auspices of a tertiary medical association. Yet in judicial practice, the People's Court initially marginalizes technical identification of medical accidents and worships judicial appraisal as a key basis for determining facts, especially after the Tort Liability Law along with the promulgation of the 2005 Decision of the Standing Committee of the National People's Congress on Issues Concerning the Management of Forensic Identification. There is no medical damage appraisal in the Tort Liability Law, making positioning the technical appraisal of medical accidents an urgent issue. Academic circles argue that flaws spread in both medical accident appraisal and medical judicial appraisal, and the dual appraisal system leads to frequent appraisals, doubling the burden on the parties and the court, hindering litigation efficiency, and

---

1 Yang Lixin, "Successes and Shortcomings in Reforming the Medical Damage Liability System under the Tort Liability Law," *Journal of Renmin University of China*, no. 4 (2010): 9.

preventing medical disputes from being resolved in a timely manner. Long before the promulgation of the Tort Liability Law, scholars analyzed the shortcomings of the "dualized" identification system and proposed a unified medical damage identification system.[1]

3. Key elements of deepening the reform of the medical and health system

"We must establish and improve the medical and health legal system, streamline medical dispute handling mechanisms, and make a mechanism for managing patient complaints and a third-party mediation mechanism for doctor-patient disputes," advocates the Opinions on Deepening the Reform of the Medical and Health System of the Central Committee of the Communist Party of China and the State Council, and the Guiding Opinions on the Pilot Reform of Public Hospitals of the Ministry of Health, the Central Administration, the National Development and Reform Commission, the Ministry of Finance, and the Ministry of Human Resources and Social Security. Proper handling of patient complaints and doctor-patient disputes has become one of the important elements of healthcare system reform.

4. Objective needs to change mindsets and medical models and explore new paths to prevent medical disputes

The issue that should be of concern is not the discord in the doctor-patient relationship, but rather that the worsening doctor-patient relationship has not improved as a result of advancing healthcare system reform, nor has it improved significantly due to the concerns of the government, hospitals, and medical personnel. In contrast, a survey by scholars showed that from 2011 to 2013, the total number of doctor-patient disputes, outpatient emergency disputes, and inpatient disputes all increased steadily year by year, up

---

1   Sun Huazhi, "Discussion on the Establishment of a Medical Assessment System," *Journal of Law and Medicine*, no. 2 (2004): 43–44.

to 55.62 doctor-patient disputes per year per medical institution.[1] Violent medical injuries in hospital settings are on the rise.[2]

Over the years, hospitals simply turned to "negative and conservative countermeasures" in "addressing such disputes." It failed to ease the doctor-patient relationship still and instead made it increasingly strained, antagonistic, alienated, and even apathetic.[3]

Modern medical education mainly comes from scientific determinism and humanism, Professor Robin believes, from the perspective of educational philosophy. It requires medical education to value not only the teaching of medical specialties but also humanities and social science education that are now jostling for attention from medical schools in developed countries throughout the entire medical education, as the "biological-psychological-social" medical model is gradually recognized. Students short of a foundation in humanities and social sciences often lose their intellectual challenges and ability to respond to such challenges during their medical careers, according to the US Training Physicians for the 21st Century, Physicians' General Professional Education (GPEP) report.[4] To this day, medical education in China still follows the biomedical education model, focusing on science over humanities. Clinicians put "treating diseases and saving people" and "disease" high on the agenda rather than "helping patients" or "patients." A cruel irony comes to the large-scale development business model of medical institutions and the "win by quantity" performance evaluation model that has further hindered the transformation of the medical model. Despite their rise with the lark early and staying up late, physicians are still incompetent to meet the needs of new Chinese patients with a resurgent sense of rights and are overwhelmed ... Changing the medical model

---

1 Yang Li, Gu Jiadong, and Jiang Baisheng, "Analysis and Countermeasures of Doctor-Patient Disputes in a Province in 2011–2013," *Journal of Nanjing Medical University (Social Science Edition)*, no. 5 (2015): 344.

2 Jia Xiaoli et al., "Research on Violent Medical Injuries in Hospitals across the Country from 2003 to 2012," *Chinese Hospitals*, no. 3 (2014): 3.

3 Wang Yue, "'Negative Protection' or 'Positive Change,'" *Chinese Hospital Director*, no. 14 (2014): 82–84.

4 Cai Fenglei et al., "A Brief Discussion on American Medical Education Reform and Its Characteristics," *Northwest Medical Education*, no. 1 (2012): 60.

is harder to get without fundamentally changing the business model and performance assessment model of medical institutions.

5. Urgent need to summarize practical experience and improve local people's mediation and physicians' liability insurance models

Since 2000, critical reflection on "litigation universalism" has continued in China. The idea that the dispute resolution mechanism must be compatible with the type of dispute is deeply rooted in people's hearts and is widely agreed upon. Attempts to establish and improve diversified dispute resolution mechanisms are also in full swing and are becoming more rational.[1] In recent years, Zhejiang, Tianjin, Shanghai, and other places have taken handling medical disputes as an important part of deepening medical and health system reform and innovating social management. Focusing on the three links of "prevention, treatment, and mediation," they have focused on constructing more scientific prevention mechanisms, more coordinated handling mechanisms, and more effective mediation mechanisms, forming a new pattern of medical dispute prevention and handling with "comprehensive management leading, departmental coordination, and professional mediation." An urgent task awaits ahead to consolidate and expand successful local experiences and achievements through legislation.

---

1   Liu Jialiang, "The Practical Model of People's Mediation in Medical Disputes and Its Implications," *Politics and Law*, no. 5 (2012): 156.

II. Legislative Principles that the Regulations on the Prevention and Handling of Medical Disputes Should Adhere To

1. Coordination and linkage principle

Medical disputes, the terminal expression of complex social problems in most cases, cannot be tackled by the sole health and family planning department. In response to conundrums that tend to occur in medical institutions, all functional departments of the local government must fulfill their duties, collaborate, and work together, and must not stand idly by and watch. Therefore, the Medical Dispute Prevention and Handling Regulations adheres to the principle of coordination and linkage. In addition to the health and family planning departments, government functional departments such as civil affairs, justice, public security, and insurance must also actively prevent and handle medical disputes to jointly build a harmonious doctor-patient relationship. The Medical Dispute Prevention and Handling Regulations should at least clarify the responsibilities of the following departments: the Health and Family Planning Department of the State Council (prevention of medical disputes, administrative identification and administrative penalties for medical accidents), the Public Security Department of the State Council (guaranteeing medical order, people's mediation order), the Civil Affairs Department of the State Council (bears the medical expenses of abandoned minor patients, elderly patients, and homeless beggars), the Judiciary Department of the State Council (People's Mediation of Medical Disputes), and the Development and Reform Department of the State Council (approval of charging standards for medical liability insurance and medical accident insurance), Insurance Regulatory Commission of the State Council (establishing and managing medical liability insurance and medical accident insurance).

2. Prevention-oriented principle

In the doctor-patient relationship, doctors naturally enjoy the dominating privilege due to their expertise, so the vast majority of medical disputes can be prevented. Therefore, the Medical Dispute Prevention and Handling Regulations adhere to the principle of prevention as the main focus, strive to pass legislation to enable medical institutions and medical personnel to establish "patient-centered" values, overcome the temptations of "egoism" ideas, strive to pass legislation to force medical institutions and medical personnel to shift from a biomedical model to a humanistic medical model, and strive to pass legislation to get medical institutions and medical personnel out of the misunderstandings of "focusing on treating patients, helping others lightly" and "focusing on technology, light on service."

3. Discriminatory response to medical negligence

Indeed, medical disputes are due to technical faults, while some are due to ethical faults. The former is often unavoidable in the careers of medical personnel, and the advancement and development of medical technology also depend on it. It is acceptable for technical factors to go wrong, but not the same mistakes. Practitioners should be encouraged to report technical mistakes in order to warn their peers. Ethical faults, on the other hand, should be strictly distinguished from technical medical negligence. For technical medical faults, heavy notification and light punishment, and those who voluntarily report should even be exempted from their administrative responsibilities; however, ethical medical negligence must not only be punished, but serious circumstances should be included in the scope of a ban on medical practitioners.

4. Fairness- and efficiency-balanced principle

Two features of medical disputes are held accountable for social incidents that evolved therefrom. First, medical disputes often involve the judgment and factual determination of medical professional issues, and due to the asymmetry of knowledge, it is impossible for patients to trust their impartiality and objectivity, whether it is a judgment made by a health administration department or an appraisal organized by a medical association. Secondly, medical dispute cases are often delayed for a long time due to identification issues. English law proverb: "Justice Delayer is justice denied. It reminds us of the problem of the prescription of justice; that is, justice itself has the connotation of prescription. Delayed justice has no real meaning; it is actually unjust for those who desire justice. Therefore, processing efficiency should be improved through third-party people's mediation mechanisms and administrative mediation mechanisms, and the fairness and objectivity of processing should be improved through a pool of consulting experts, mainly medical experts.

5. Social sharing of medical risks

A limited understanding of human laws makes medical treatment a highly dangerous act. There are only two ways to avoid personal harm to patients: "reduce the number of actions" or "transfer risk."[1] Medical institutions must reduce the number of unnecessary medical practices and avoid excessive medical treatment, but refusing to implement necessary medical practices because of risk is clearly contrary to the medical value orientation of maximizing the interests of patients. Therefore, transferring risk is a reasonable way to avoid personal harm due to medical practices.[2]

III. Key Issue 1: Whether to Maintain the Concept of Medical Malpractice

Representatives of health administration departments proposed the complete abolition of the concept of medical accidents in drafting the Medical Dispute Prevention and Handling Regulations (Draft for Review). The author votes for maintaining the concept of medical accidents. First, although

---

1   Zheng Bingwen, "The Welfare State in Economic Theory," *Chinese Social Science*, no. 1 (2003): 41–43.

2   Wang Yue, "Reflecting on Legal Issues in Clinical Drug Trials in China from the 'Korean Ginseng Pill Incident," *Chinese Pharmacy*, no. 5 (2005): 4–7.

with the implementation of the Tort Liability Law, people's courts no longer refer to the Regulations on Medical Accident Treatment, apply the concept of medical accidents, and have begun to use medical damage compensation or medical service contract disputes as the cause of the case, the concept of medical malpractice should continue to exist, which should return to its original administrative law function. In fact, the 2002 Regulations on Medical Accident Treatment are administrative regulations formulated and promulgated by the State Council when the National People's Congress did not issue special legislation on civil compensation for medical disputes. Therefore, its original function was to legislate on administrative legal relationships between medical institutions, medical personnel, and administrative departments. Still, it was "helplessly" given the function of adjusting civil legal relationships between medical institutions, medical personnel, and patients. The legal system for handling medical incidents must continue to exist as an important legal system for the administrative administration of medical institutions and medical personnel by administrative authorities, and along with the reform of separation of administration and administration, this system should play a more important role in the future. Second, only by retaining the concept of medical malpractice can it be legally connected with the crime of medical malpractice in Article 335 of the Criminal Law. Otherwise, serious medical damage incidents that cause serious personal injury to patients will not be investigated for criminal liability. There is confusion and failure in the application of the law.

It is important to note here that medical accidents defined by the Medical Dispute Prevention and Handling Regulations and medical damage defined in the Tort Liability Law are different. If following the previous four elements of medical accidents, it is said that medical damage should be examined (in fact, the Tort Liability Law has changed the subjective fault judgment to the current objective fault judgment, that is, ignoring the judgment of motives and paying attention to the examination of the duty of care standard, so most scholars think it is the three elements). The difference between the two is shown in Table 1.

Table 1. Comparison of medical accidents and medical damage

	Medical malpractice	Medical damage
Illegality requirements	Violate medical and health management laws, administrative regulations, departmental rules, diagnosis, treatment, and nursing standards and routines	Medical personnel did not fulfill their medical obligations corresponding to the level of medical treatment at the time in diagnosis and treatment activities
Fault element	Negligence	Negligence or intentional fault
Outcome requirements	Causing personal damage to the patient (right to life, right to health, and right to health)	Cause damage to the patient's personal rights (right to life, right to health, right to health, right to name, right to image, right to reputation, right to chastity, right to privacy, etc.) and property rights
Causation	Absolute causation	Quite a causal relationship

Since medical accidents have returned to their administrative law functions, their scope should differ from the medical damage boundary of civil liability. That is, what constitutes a medical injury does not necessarily constitute a medical accident. Medical disputes, on the other hand, have the broadest meaning and extension. Currently, they are described as disputes between medical institutions, their medical personnel, and patients due to medical services such as medical treatment and nursing. Figure 1 clearly shows the logical relationship between medical disputes, medical damage (civil liability), and medical accidents (administrative or criminal liability).

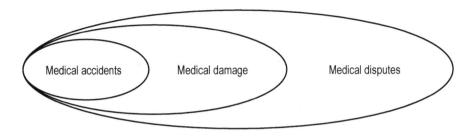

Figure 1. Relationship between medical accidents, medical damage,
and medical disputes

IV. Key Issue 2: Innovative Mechanisms for Medical Dispute Prevention

The biggest problem with the Medical Dispute Prevention and Handling Regulations (Draft for Review) is that the legislation does not focus on prevention. Instead, it puts a lot of space on handling. From the name of the law, it can be seen that prevention should be placed in an important position. The author wants to legalize the following innovations in medical dispute prevention mechanisms.

1. Gradually abolish outpatient clinics in tertiary hospitals and clearly limit the work intensity standards for medical staff

One of the goals of healthcare system reform is to achieve hierarchical diagnosis and treatment, so that patients with common diseases and chronic diseases can be reduced to primary medical institutions. However, there is a direct relationship between the quality of work of medical personnel and the work intensity of medical personnel.[1] If it is not possible to fundamentally limit the motivation of medical institutions to seek profit and correct the

---

1   Zhang Zheng and Gao Jie, "A Study on the Influence of the Work Intensity of Medical Personnel on the Quality Level of Medical Care," *Southwest Defense Pharmaceutical*, no. 5 (2010): 561.

fact that medical personnel are currently working too hard, it will be diffi-cult to resolve medical disputes completely.

Legislative Suggestions

Article XX [Hierarchical Diagnosis and Treatment System and Maximum Work Intensity System for Medical Personnel]

The health and family planning department under the State Council should formulate an implementation plan to gradually abolish outpatient clinics in tertiary medical institutions, and formulate specific quantitative indicators to evaluate the maximum work intensity of medical personnel at medical institutions at all levels, guide the rational diversion of patients, and prohibit medical institutions from being overloaded or overworked.

In case of overloaded medical institutions and work intensity, medical staff have the right to file a complaint through a trade union or health administration department and seek improvements.

---

2. Ban on revenue generation indicators was upgraded to a legal requirement

The National Health and Family Planning Commission has issued three orders and five declarations strictly prohibiting medical institutions from issuing economic indicators to departments, and directly linking the income of medical staff to the economic income of departments. However, medical institutions changed the economic income index of departments to the index of workload linked to the income of medical personnel; in fact, they changed soup instead of medicine. As an administrative regulation, the Medical Dispute Prevention and Handling Regulations clarifies violators' legal responsibilities and strives to reverse the "work more, gain more" in hospitals to "work hard and get well."

Legislative Suggestions

Article XX [Benefits for Medical Personnel]

It is strictly prohibited for medical institutions to issue economic indicators to departments, and it is strictly prohibited to directly link the income of medical personnel to the department's financial income or the workload of medical staff. Medical institutions should ensure that medical personnel have good benefits and purchase corresponding insurance for medical personnel in special positions. Medical institutions shall ensure that the benefits of emergency and pediatric medical personnel are not lower than those of other departments."

3. Improve the effectiveness of the work of medical service quality control departments and complaint consultation departments

Currently, the hospital's medical service quality monitoring department often does not get the understanding and cooperation of the clinical departments. It becomes a formality, coping with things, and even the management and clinical medical staff go their own way.[1] Clinical experts must be gradually trained into managers through systems and become the backbone of hospital management. In addition, the current complaints department generally has a problematic positioning, making patients feel that they are standing on the hospital's side. If patients can vent their dissatisfaction with medical staff in a timely manner, it will help avoid vicious medical disputes in the future.

---

1   Liu Yu and Chen Wei, "Historical Progress and Future Prospects of Hospital Complaint Management," *Chinese Hospitals*, no. 6 (2011): 67–68.

Legislative Suggestions

Article XX [Medical Service Quality Control Department and Complaint Consultation Department]

A medical institution shall establish a medical service quality control department, which is specifically responsible for supervising the medical service work of the medical personnel and checking the medical personnel's practice.

Medical institutions should set up a medical service complaint consultation department to be specifically responsible for accepting various complaints from patients or family members against medical staff and consultation related to medical services. If a patient or family member needs to continue treatment after complaining to a medical staff member, the medical institution must replace the medical staff for the patient. Medical institutions above the county level must set up a 24-hour consultation desk or consultation hotline, and a special person is responsible for answering inquiries related to medical services.

The head of the medical institution must also serve as the head of the medical service quality control department and assume the primary responsibility for the quality of the medical service in the medical institution. The head of the clinical department of a medical institution must work exclusively (part-time) for at least half a year in the medical service quality control department and complaints department."

4. Change the concept of service and add non-revenue-generating departments and locations

Over the years, there have been many cases of serious medical injuries and murders that have received national attention. Investigations by academics show that most of the vicious wounded have a low level of education, with poor families, the unemployed, farmers, and laid-off workers accounting for more than 70%; nearly 40% are introverted, isolated, and paranoid, and nearly 30% have a history of mental illness; and there are also phenomena such as untreatable diseases and difficulties in paying medical expenses. Therefore, medical institutions must shift the center of work from "disease" to "people," and overcome the influence of utilitarianism on us to meet the requirements of a period of social transformation. Medical institutions should set up "medical social worker departments" and "psychological counseling departments" and pay special attention to special services for the disabled, the elderly, children, pregnant women, foreigners, and people from ethnic minorities. Medical institutions at or above the county level should provide life assistance to patients as much as possible, including but not limited to setting up mother and child rooms, prayer rooms for ethnic minority patients or people with religious beliefs, play areas for children, and farewell rooms.

Legislative Suggestions

Article XX [Medical Social Work Department]

Medical institutions at or above the county level shall set up medical social worker departments, which are specifically responsible for recruiting, training, and organizing public members to participate in the hospital's medical social worker work. Medical social workers should be mainly recruited from the community, and at the same time, young medical personnel in medical institutions should be encouraged as a supplement.

Medical social work departments should strengthen communication with medical personnel to understand patients' financial capabilities. For patients with financial difficulties, medical social work departments must pay special attention to their lives; for some patients with special difficulties, medical social work departments should raise funds from the community through media, charitable organizations, etc., to help poor patients in medical institutions.

Article XX [Psychological Counseling Department]

Medical institutions at or above the county level shall set up psychological counseling departments, and clinical psychologists or psychological counselors shall provide psychological counseling services to patients. Clinical psychologists or counselors should participate in the hospital's administrative inspection and propose psychological intervention suggestions and plans for patients with psychological problems.

Clinical psychologists or counselors shall provide free psychological counseling services to medical staff in this hospital.

Article XX [Life Assistance for Special Patients]

Medical institutions at or above the county level must establish special services for the disabled, the elderly, children, pregnant women, foreigners, and ethnic minority people to resolve their difficulties. Medical institutions at or above the county level should provide life assistance to patients as much as possible, including but not limited to setting up mother and child rooms, prayer rooms for minority patients or people with religious beliefs, play areas for children, and farewell rooms.

5. Closed management of emergency areas

Emergency departments are also departments with frequent medical disputes. According to the characteristics of emergency departments and the unity of interests of patients, families, and emergency physicians, the Medical Dispute Prevention and Handling Regulations make it clear that medical institutions at or above the county level should implement closed management of emergency areas. To obtain rescue time, medical institutions can obtain authorization from patients' families through alternative consent methods such as emergency patient authorization letters to rescue patients in the best interests of patients.

Legislative Suggestions

Article XX [Emergency Care Dispute Prevention]

Medical institutions at or above the county level shall implement closed management of emergency areas. In order to obtain rescue time, medical institutions can obtain authorization from patients' families through alternative consent methods such as emergency patient authorization letters to rescue patients in the best interests of patients.

---

6. Informed consent recording inspection system for major surgeries, special patients with poor understanding ability, and experimental medical behavior

Progress in society and the spread of Internet technology proliferate "learning patients." More importantly, the patriarchal doctor-patient relationship no longer answers to the requirements of patients. They strongly demand participation in clinical decision-making and sharing expertise in "condition, treatment options, risks, and costs" with medical staff. The only way to avoid disputes is to share professional knowledge and ultimately reach a consensus. However, over the years, the "informed consent" system in China's medical industry has focused on "consent" during the implementation process. As a result, "sign it" has become a clinical mantra, mistakenly believed that the "informed consent" system relieves hospitals of all responsibilities. Hence, informed consent has much resemblance to a "statement of life and death," with exemptions from liability running from the first to the last clause, leaving patients with no medical knowledge discouraged and afraid to sign. In fact, the "informed consent" system introduced by Western society should focus on "acknowledge" rather than "consent," as consent without acknowledgment or understanding is legally invalid. Only an expression of true meaning based on understanding can make physicians' professional conduct a deterrent but illegal matter. Even if you have legally passed the "patient has understood the above content" exemption clause to try to remove your responsibilities, the patient will definitely be unforgiving to the physician due to differences in perception before and after surgery.[1]

There are many areas where hospitals need to improve when it comes to informed consent. First, the informed consent form prepared by the medical institution should be made in two copies. After the patient or close family member signs it, hand it over to them for preservation in one copy to avoid unnecessary suspicions and misunderstandings. Second, most vicious medical disputes are related to surgery, and the content of informed consent is often the most concentrated part of the dispute between the parties to the dispute. Instead of treating informed consent prior to surgery, special tests, and treatment as an exemption from liability or a measure of self-protection, healthcare workers should value informed consent as a process of educating patients. Physicians should make full use of various forms, such as anatomical maps, anatomical models, and multimedia courseware, and use language that patients can understand to interact with patients. Second, medical institutions at or above the county level should implement a hierarchical management system for surgeries and record the entire conversation for "four-level surgeries," "special patients with poor understanding," and "experimental medical behaviors" for future reference, to avoid future factual disputes. Also, it forces medical staff to pay attention to the authenticity and objectivity of what they tell patients.

---

1 Wang Yue, "Is Informed Consent a 'Legal Exemption' or a 'Consensus Reached,'" *Chinese Medical Humanities*, no. 2 (2015): 43.

Legislative Suggestions

Article XX [Informed Consent]

When a medical institution performs surgery, special examination, or special treatment, it must obtain the patient's consent; when it is unable to obtain the patient's opinion, it should obtain the consent and signature of a close family member.

The informed consent form prepared by the medical institution should be made in two copies. After the patient or close family member signs it, hand it over to them for preservation.

Article XX [Purpose and Method of Informed Consent]

Instead of treating informed consent prior to surgery, special tests, and treatment as an exemption from liability or a measure of self-protection, healthcare workers should value informed consent as a process of educating patients. Physicians should make full use of various forms such as anatomical maps, anatomical models, multimedia courseware, etc., and languages that patients can understand to interact with patients.

When patients need to make decisions about their treatment, physicians should communicate with them in an interactive manner as much as possible and answer their questions as much as possible.

Article XX [Informed Consent Recording System for Major Surgery and Experimental Medical Practices]

Medical institutions at or above the county level should implement a hierarchical surgical management system. For level 4 surgeries, special patients with poor understanding ability, and experimental medical practices, the medical service quality control department should be responsible for organizing both physicians and patients

> to carry out pre-operative notifications. After obtaining the patient's
> consent, the entire conversation will be recorded for inspection.

7. Alternative consent and pre-life prediction system

Medical disputes also often arise overprotective treatment measures for special patients, such as cancer and life-sustaining treatment for terminally ill
patients. Although the "Shenzhen Wen Yuzhang extortion and murder of
his wife," which is a national sensation, finally found Wen Yuzhang guilty of
intentional homicide and sentenced to three years in prison and suspended
for three years.[1] There are shuddering cases that are far from proceeding to
judicial review on a daily basis. In recent years, civil society organizations
on death with dignity in mainland China have made certain efforts in this
regard, objectively promoting the development of death with dignity. For
example, in May 2009, the "Choice and Dignity" charity website published
the first folk text, "My Five Wishes" (i.e., what medical services do I want or
don't want; I want to use or not use life support treatment; how I want others
to treat me; what I want my family and friends to know; who I want to help
me). It hopes to let more people know what "Predicting My Life" means and
how to use "Predicting Life" to pre-dispose the risks they may face when
they die. However, the activities of such civil society organizations are more
about educating the public about death and publicizing death. We should
pass the State Council's legislation to resolve the difficult issues for both clinicians and patients' families. For example, Singapore's "Advance Medical
Instructions Act" stipulates that advance medical instructions are attached
to the patient's medical records. Medical personnel are only allowed to

---

1   Guo Biao, "The Second Trial in the Shenzhen Extortion of His Wife Was Handed Down
    Today," *Nanfang Daily*, September 14, 2012.

check whether patients have signed advance medical instructions when they fall into a coma.[1]

Legislative Suggestions

Article XX [Alternate Consent and Pre-life Probation System]

Medical personnel should treat terminally ill patients' choices of life-sustaining treatment with care. Respecting the wishes expressed by incapacitated patients before they became incapacitated can protect patients' right to make autonomous decisions to the greatest extent possible through methods such as living wills and alternative consent.

---

8. New functions of the Medical Ethics Committee: access to new technology and punishment of ethical damage

From "vagus nerve detachment and fixation for rheumatoid arthritis treatment" to "broken limb lengthening surgery," from "electric shock withdrawal from internet addiction" to "surgical drug rehabilitation" to the "Wei Zexi Incident" which recently caused a national stir, scandals caused by clinical misuse of new technology have had the credibility of the medical industry severely damaged time and time again. However, in 2015, in accordance with the State Council's Decision on Cancelling Non-administrative License Approval Matters, the State Health Planning Commission canceled the approval for clinical application of Class III medical technology and abolished the Catalogue of the First Batch of Class III Medical Technology Allowed for Clinical Application issued on May 22, 2009. The third type of medical technology in this catalog includes 19 types of allogeneic organ transplantation

---

1   Luo Diandian, *Who Is in Charge of My Death* (Beijing: Writers Publishing House, 2011), 18.

technology, denaturation technology, and gene chip diagnosis technology. This is bound to cause the entry of new clinical technology to present a management vacuum. However, under special conditions, unproven therapies can be used as experimental treatments for patients when certain conditions are met. Still, experimental treatment must meet certain conditions and be limited to a small number of patients. Medical institutions at or above the county level shall establish medical ethics committees as the highest authority for making medical clinical technical decisions. Administrative management cadres of medical institutions are prohibited from holding positions on medical ethics committees and are not allowed to interfere with the work of medical ethics committees.

Legislative Suggestions

Article XX [Medical Ethics Committee]

Medical institutions at or above the county level shall establish medical ethics committees as the highest authority for making medical clinical technical decisions. Administrative management cadres of medical institutions are not allowed to hold positions on the Medical Ethics Committee and must not interfere with the work of the Medical Ethics Committee. Specific measures shall be separately formulated by the Health and Family Planning Department under the State Council.

The Medical Ethics Committee is responsible for making decisions on the following issues relating to clinical technology:

(1) Experimental medical behavior issues
(2) The issue of clinical admission to new technologies
(3) Drug use problems that exceed registration information
(4) Internal review issues of medical errors
(5) Punishment issues for ethical medical errors
(6) Other issues related to clinical technology

---

9. Avoiding medical disputes arising from medical records

There are not a few medical disputes arising from medical records. First, there should be no longer any distinction between subjective medical records and objective medical records. The Regulations on Medical Accident Treatment stipulate that patients can only copy objective medical records and that subjective medical records are sealed in the presence of both parties. The distinction between subjective medical records and objective medical records in practice artificially creates conflicts and disputes between doctors and patients and increases patients' distrust of hospitals. If a medical dispute enters the judicial process, subjective medical records must also be provided to patients, so the Medical Dispute Prevention and Handling Regulations should no longer discriminate between subjective and objective medical records.

Legislative Suggestions

Article XX [Retention, Reproduction, and Archiving of Medical Records]

Medical institutions shall properly keep patient inpatient medical records and patient outpatient (emergency) medical records kept by medical institutions.

Medical institutions should implement a 24-hour medical records filing system. Patients or their close relatives need to copy medical records from 24 hours ago. The medical institution should provide all medical records, draw up a list, and stamp the certificate. Medical institutions must not refuse to provide copies of medical records on the grounds that patients have not completed discharge procedures.

If a patient or their close relatives request that medical records or physical objects be sealed, both physician-patient parties shall jointly carry out the sealing. Where medical records or physical

> objects are sealed on site, the medical institution shall draw up a
> sealed list, which shall be kept one copy after being sealed or signed
> by both parties concerned.

10. Humanistic care for the deceased

When a patient dies, it is often a period of emotional turbulence for the family. At this time, medical staff often do not pay attention to humanistic care for the patient's family, which in turn may cause dissatisfaction that has been saved for a long time to erupt once upon the patient's death. Therefore, legislation should focus on the issue of humanistic care for deceased patients.

Legislative Suggestions

Article XX [Human Care for Deceased Patients]

Medical institutions at or above the county level shall set up end-of-life farewell rooms. If a patient dies in a medical institution, the medical institution shall send the corpse to the final farewell room, and the medical social worker department shall organize the family to say goodbye to the patient at the end of life, then move it to the morgue, and inform them of the specific steps for follow-up matters such as burial."

V. Key Issue 3: Whether to Maintain Administrative Processing and Administrative Mediation as Remedies for Medical Disputes

The Regulations on Medical Accident Treatment establish three remedies: settlement, administrative processing, and judicial processing. Based on the experience of people's mediation in medical disputes in various regions, the Medical Dispute Prevention and Handling Regulations (Draft for Review) added one form of relief on this basis, that is, people's mediation, but abolished the original administrative handling and administrative mediation of the administrative departments of healthcare. The author believes that in the face of the current poor handling of medical disputes, the means of relief "should be increased rather than reduced," and considering administrative functions of health and family planning departments, especially their professional characteristics in handling medical disputes, administrative handling and administrative mediation should still be preserved. If patients trust the health administrative department, especially with the promotion of separate administration and administration, relief channels for patients to quickly handle medical disputes through administrative authorities should be preserved.

Legislative Suggestions

Article XX [Means of Handling Medical Disputes]

After a medical dispute occurs, both the doctor and the patient can choose the following ways to resolve it:
  (1) Negotiate on your own
  (2) Apply to the People's Mediation Committee for Medical Disputes for People's Mediation
  (3) Apply to the health and family planning department for administrative processing
  (4) Bring a lawsuit to the people's court

VI. Key Issue 4: Medical Accident Technical Assessment Should Return to Administrative Assessment

At present, there is a dual-track phenomenon of judicial appraisal and medical association technical appraisal in civil trials of medical disputes, and people's courts often use the appraisal conclusions of judicial appraisal as the basis for determining cases. From the trend of judicial reform, first of all, the competent departments of appraisal opinions needed by the people's courts to find out the facts in the trial of cases have been included in the judicial appraisal system of the Ministry of Justice, while the appraisal of medical associations will inevitably be marginalized if it is not included in the judicial appraisal system; Secondly, according to the legislative trend of the new Civil Procedure Law, "judicial expertise conclusion" has been renamed as "judicial expertise opinion," so "one appraisal is final" in China's judicial trial will also become history. Since the Regulations on Medical Accident Treatment establishes a complete medical accident technical assessment system, it is recommended to retain it and return it to its proper function, that is, to position it as an administrative assessment, as an assessment procedure entrusted by the health and family planning department to determine whether it constitutes a medical incident and whether administrative punishment should be imposed.

Legislative Suggestions

Article XX [Commencement of Technical Assessment of Medical Malpractice]

After receiving a medical accident dispute, the administrative department of public health, in addition to ordering the medical institution to promptly take necessary medical treatment measures to prevent the consequences of damage from spreading, shall orga-

---

nize an investigation to determine whether it is a medical accident; if it is unable to determine whether it is a medical accident, it shall submit it to the medical association responsible for the technical assessment of the medical accident to organize an assessment in accordance with the relevant provisions of these Regulations.

VII. Key Issue 5: Restoring the Classification of Responsible Medical Incidents and Technical Medical Incidents

The Regulations on the Handling of Medical Accidents cancel the distinction between responsible medical accidents and technical medical accidents in the Measures for the Handling of Medical Accidents, and they are collectively referred to as medical accidents. In practice, this has been found to be problematic. First, due to the high-risk nature of medical technology, it is very difficult for medical personnel not to make technical mistakes. On the contrary, technical negligence helps to learn from experience and advance the development of medical technology, so the classification of responsible and technical accidents in medical accidents should be restored. Heavy penalties for responsible accidents and even a lifelong ban on employment (should be linked to the revision of the Medical Practitioners Law); heavy sharing of technical accidents can be exempted from administrative penalties. Secondly, the failure to define responsible medical and technical medical malpractice makes it difficult to identify the crime of medical malpractice in the Criminal Law and even leads to abuse of judicial power. Only by restoring responsible medical malpractice and technical medical malpractice can judicial power be effectively regulated by professional judgment.

Legislative Suggestions

Article XX [Classification of Medical Errors]

Medical accidents are divided into accidents and technical accidents. An accident of responsibility refers to a medical accident caused by a medical worker's dereliction of duty, such as violating rules and regulations, diagnosis, treatment, and nursing routines due to a lack of sense of responsibility; a technical accident refers to a medical accident caused by a medical staff member's lack of experience. Technical accidents are not subject to administrative penalties.

Medical institutions and medical personnel who report a technical accident to the health and family planning department of the people's government at the county level are exempt from administrative punishment, and their report shall not be used as evaluation evidence for the medical institution's quality control standards."

VIII. Key Issue 6: Urgent Need to Establish a Supplementary Medical Accident Insurance System

According to the spirit of civil law, civil remedies should be obtained if there is damage, regardless of whether there is a fault or not. We can summarize the causes of social damage into two categories: one is called an "unlawful act," and the second is called an "unfortunate incident," However, the Medical Dispute Prevention and Handling Regulations (Draft for Review) only mentions the medical liability insurance system and omits the medical accident insurance system. In reality, the latter is more important than the former for easing the doctor-patient relationship, especially with regard to medical accidents where no one party is at fault. This is exactly the reason for many protracted medical incidents. A complete medical dispute insurance system should include two aspects: on the one hand, medical liability insurance allows primary medical institutions not to affect their economic operations due to huge civil compensation for "illegal" personal injury; on the other hand, through medical accident insurance, patients who have performed high-risk surgeries and examinations can receive financial compensation that makes them more satisfied once "unfortunate" personal damage occurs. Over the years, some of the top three medical institutions have made very useful explorations in this area.[1] Since medical accident insurance should not be fully rolled out, it should start with high-risk medical service projects. It is recommended that the health, family planning, development, reform, and insurance supervision departments of the provincial people's governments should regularly publish and adjust the "Compulsory Medical Accident Insurance Catalogue for High-Risk Medical Service Projects" according to local conditions, add medical accident insurance benefits to high-risk medical service projects included in the catalog, and establish a provincial medical accident insurance fund.

Legislative Suggestions

Article XX [Medical Liability Insurance System]

The health and family planning departments of provincial people's governments should encourage medical institutions to participate in medical liability insurance and establish provincial medical liability insurance funds.

Underwriters are encouraged to participate in the quality management of medical services in medical institutions.

---

1 Wang Weidong, Li Wenbin, and Lin Fangfang, "Implementing Medical Accident Insurance to Create a Harmonious Doctor-Patient Relationship," *China's Health Law System* 25, no. 2 (2017): 68.

Article XX [Medical Accident Insurance System]

Medical accidents are the risk costs of medical services. The health and family planning, development and reform, and insurance supervisory departments of the provincial people's governments shall regularly publish and adjust the Catalogue of Compulsory Medical Accident Insurance for High-Risk Medical Service Projects in accordance with local conditions, add medical accident insurance benefits to high-risk medical service items included in the catalog, and establish a provincial medical accident insurance fund."

Comparative Allocation of Burden of Proof for Extraterritorial Medical Damage and China's Strategy

I. Concept and Meaning of the Burden of Proof

The concept of burden of proof originates from Roman law. The provisions of Roman law on the burden of proof system can be summarized in five sentences: "The plaintiff's right to his lawsuit, and his claim must be proved by proof," "If the plaintiff does not prove it, the defendant wins the case," "If a defense is raised, then there is a need to prove his defense," "The person making the claim has no obligation to prove it, but the person who denies it," and "Due to the nature of the matter, the person who denies it does not need to prove it." In German law, "Beweislast" is used to express the burden of proof. Japan draws on German doctrine and translates "Beweislast" in German law as "burden of proof," "burden of proof," and "burden of proof." At the end of the Qing Dynasty, the term burden of proof was introduced from Japan to China. The original meaning was "who argues and who gives proof," that is, the parties should bear the responsibility of providing evidence for their own claims; otherwise, they will bear unfavorable litigation results.

It can be seen that as early as Roman law, the burden of proof confirmed two basic principles: one is that "the plaintiff has the burden of proof," which is a reflection of the ancient law "without a plaintiff, no official" in the law of evidence; the second is that "there is no obligation to prove for those who make claims, nothing for those who deny," that is, "those who affirm should bear the burden of proof, and those who deny it have no burden of proof." The burden of proof system at the time was already quite complete, and this established the "who claims, who gives evidence" certification rule, which had a huge impact on future generations. In the process of long-term theoretical exploration and trial practice, people have also continuously developed the meaning of the burden of proof and formed various theories. The burden of proof has different connotations in different historical periods, and the two major legal systems have different understandings of it. However, "burden of proof" as a legal term has been widely used.

In civil law systems, the term "burden of proof" has two meanings: first, when a party has a claim in a lawsuit, they must submit relevant evidence to support their claim; otherwise, they will suffer an unfavorable outcome, which is called the "subjective burden of proof"; second, at the end of the lawsuit, when the existence of certain facts is still uncertain, one of the parties is at risk of being judged unfavorably by the court, called the "objective burden of proof." Currently, the "burden of proof" commonly used in Germany and Japan mostly refers to the "objective burden of proof."

English and American law scholars believe that the burden of proof includes two meanings: the responsibility to provide evidence and the burden of persuasion. "The responsibility to provide evidence" refers to "the responsibility to provide evidence on the disputed facts at the beginning of litigation, or at any stage of trial or debate." This is a behavioral responsibility of the parties. If the parties fail to fulfill their responsibility to provide evidence, The case shall not be submitted to the jury for consideration, and the judge shall directly rule against the person responsible for providing evidence. "The burden of persuasion" means that "a party who bears this specific burden bears the risk of any disputed fact that he has asserted—if he cannot conclusively prove his assertion, he will lose the case." This is for cases that have been handed over to the jury for deliberation. At the end of the evidence investigation, if the jury is still unable to determine the truth or falsehood of the disputed facts, the party with specific liability will bear the litigation disadvantages caused by this.

The current understanding and expression of the burden of proof by the legal community in China is the "double meaning statement" is currently a common statement. According to this statement, the burden of proof is dual. It includes not only who provides evidence to prove the facts of the case, but also who bears the legal consequences of not being able to provide evidence to prove the facts of the case. Responsibility for action and responsibility for results are inseparable. The "dual meaning statement" can reflect the inevitable link between the parties' proof and the lawsuit's purpose, that is, combined with the lawsuit's outcome, and the explanation of the legal nature of the burden of proof can be convincing. Article 2 of the Certain Provisions on Evidence in Civil Litigation issued by the Supreme People's Court on December 21, 2001, stipulates: "The parties concerned are responsible for providing evidence to prove the facts on which their lawsuit is based or the facts on which the other party's lawsuit is based. Where there is no evidence or evidence insufficient to prove the factual claims of the parties, the party responsible for proof shall bear the adverse consequences." This provision formally clearly defines the dual meaning of the burden of proof.

II. Allocation of the Burden of Proof

The distribution of the burden of proof refers to the parties' respective responsibilities for providing evidence for their own litigation claims in accordance with the fixed distribution rules and the time limit requirements for which the party bears the burden of proof stipulated in the law. The distribution of the burden of proof is an externalization of the nature of the burden of proof and a manifestation of its function. Its significance lies in the fact that the law stipulates which party will bear the risk of adverse litigation consequences when the truth of the facts is unknown. Therefore, it has guidance. The function of judges is to make correct decisions.

1. The principle of allocating the burden of proof in civil law

The principle of allocation of the burden of proof already existed in the Roman law era. At that time, two principles were defined for the distribution of the burden of proof. One was "the plaintiff should bear the obligation to prove," and the other was "the person making the claim has an obligation to prove, and the person who denies it has no obligation to prove." These two principles actually talk about the subjective burden of proof and the burden of providing evidence. In the early days of Roman law, people did not have the concept of objective burden of proof. Judges did not need to consider who should bear the adverse consequences when the truth of the facts to be proved was unknown. With the development of the times, these two principles are not sufficiently detailed in theory, and the exceptions to the allocation of the burden of proof that continues to occur cannot be decided based on this principle, so scholars have separated different theories to solve the problem of assigning the burden of proof. Among them, the classification of German legal elements plays an important role as a civil law country's general statement on the principle of allocating the burden of proof. The classification of legal elements is a theory that allocates the burden of proof based on the different types of legal elements stipulated in substantive law. The most influential and long-standing dominant doctrine in litigation theory is Normentheorie, which German scholar Rosenbeck founded at age 21 and became famous for publishing *Die Beweislast*. According to the regulations, according to the wording, structure, and order of application of the law, legal provisions are divided into rights based on regulations, rights obstruction provisions, rights extinguishing provisions, and prevention of the exercise of rights, and regulations that prevent the exercise of rights, and are based on the classification provided by law, and the burden of proof is distributed based on the principles and exceptions stipulated by law and the relationship between basic provisions and contrary provisions.

Simply put, the general principle of assigning the burden of proof is that "each party must assert and prove a legal norm that is beneficial to itself (equal to a regulation whose effect is favorable to itself)." This standardized method of assigning the burden of proof is simple, easy to implement, and highly operable. During the trial, judges can directly analyze the civil law provisions that should be applied and then directly apply the formula to determine where the burden of proof is distributed, so it is highly respected in trial practice. In addition to this, the regulation says that although there is no clear distinction between subjective burden of proof and objective burden of proof, it unifies responsibility for result with responsibility for action and places responsibility for results on those with unfavorable behavioral responsibility, which is in line with the essential meaning of responsibility, and requires that each party should be responsible for their own litigation actions. Its strict logical proof system has profoundly impacted the theory of burden of proof allocation. Up to now, it is still the theoretical basis for scholarly research.

However, regulations focus on the external form of legal regulation, do not pay attention to the content of legal norms, cannot properly distribute from the standpoint of legal value theory, and cannot fully estimate the fairness and justice between the parties. Therefore, the results of allocating the burden of proof based on this statement often cannot obtain substantial fairness. In particular, with the development of large industries, there are more and more damage incidents such as environmental pollution, medical disputes, traffic accidents, and product defects. For these many types of complex disputes, if we want to obtain real fairness in the distribution of the burden of proof, it seems impossible to classify the legal elements; it is necessary to reconsider the new standards for allocating the burden of proof. As a result, many scholars have proposed a new theory of the burden of proof, mainly in dangerous areas.

2. Principles for allocating the burden of proof in Anglo-American law

In Anglo-American law countries, case law has an extremely important legal status. Unlike the civil law system, the English and American law systems place importance on the lawmaking role of judges in specific cases. Therefore, although there are some theories on the allocation of the burden of proof in modern times, there are not as many opinions as in the civil law system, forming a far-reaching general applicable principle. According to the current American standard for assigning the burden of proof, there is no general standard for allocating the burden of proof; individual decisions can only be made based on the specific circumstances of the case on the basis of combining a number of allocation criteria. In other words, it is to weigh various interests and analyze specific issues in detail. For this reason, civil law scholars have summarized the modern American theory of distributing the burden of proof as a "measurement of interests theory." In summary, American scholars believe that the main factors in allocating the burden of proof are (1) policy, (2) fairness, (3) evidence holding (proof) or distance of evidence, (4) convenience, (5) probability, (6) rules of experience (ordinary human experience), and (7) the party requesting a change in the status quo should bear the burden of proof, etc. Although scholars have some differences in analyzing the decisive influence of the various factors mentioned above on the allocation of the burden of proof, they agree that the distribution of the burden of proof should be measured by integrating the three elements of policy, fairness, and probability.

The distribution of the burden of proof discussed in Anglo-American law also mainly refers to the allocation of the "burden of persuasion." As can be seen from the above explanation, civil law scholars such as Germany and Japan divide the burden of proof into "subjective burden of proof" and "objective burden of proof." In contrast, English and American law scholars divide the burden of proof into the "responsibility to provide evidence" and the "responsibility to persuade." Although the litigation model, evidence system, and trial organization of the two major legal systems are very different, scholars in the two major legal systems agree on their understanding of the burden of proof. The "burden of proof" in English and American law systems is equivalent to the "subjective burden of proof" in the civil law system, while the "burden of persuasion" of the former is equivalent to the "objective burden of proof" of the latter. This dual distinction between the two major legal systems has similar significance. The former generally refers to the obligation of the parties to provide evidence to the court after making a claim in a lawsuit in accordance with the requirements of the principle of dialecticalism; the latter means that after providing evidence, the parties concerned must bear the adverse consequences of losing the lawsuit if they do not make the judge sincerely convinced of the facts.

This theory differs from general application rules that civil law scholars have always hoped to create. It focuses on revealing the nature of the burden of proof rather than being limited to the formal elements of legal norms. It basically reflects the burden of proof that parties bear under different circumstances in trial practice and is conducive to guiding litigation practice.

The two major legal systems pursue the same purpose in distributing the burden of proof, and the highest ideal they pursue is to achieve legal fairness and justice. The difference between the two is mainly caused by differences in litigation methodology. The Anglo-American law system uses factual litigation, emphasizes the role of judges in making laws, and uses "interest measurement" as the theoretical basis for allocating the burden of proof. Although flexible, it is also arbitrary and inconsistent. The civil law system uses law-driven litigation. According to the triptych of adjudication, it emphasizes the role of judges in implementing and confirming the law in litigation and pursues lawmaking as the principle of adjudication. Therefore, its rules for assigning the burden of proof are attached to substantive regulations, have clear standards, and have the advantage of being easy to operate and reconcile with substantive law, but flexibility is clearly insufficient.

III. Allocation of the Burden of Proof in Extraterritorial Medical Disputes

1. The United States

The allocation of the burden of proof for medical damage in US law follows the "facts tell yourself" principle (Res Ipsa Loquitur). the word Res Ipsa Loquitur comes from Latin, and the English interpretation is that the thing speaks for itself, so the Chinese interpretation is self-evident, or "facts speak for themselves." The "tell yourself the facts" principle is officially used to determine tort liability. It first appeared in an infringement case heard by the English Treasury in 1863. Since the 19th century, the "show yourself" principle has been quite effective in the field of proof of fault in English and American law. To date, 34 states in the US have successfully applied the "state yourself" principle in medical damages lawsuits to reduce the burden of proof for plaintiffs.

As the problem of unjust distribution of the burden of proof between physicians and patients becomes more and more serious, courts tend to apply the principle of "explain oneself with facts" in medical lawsuits based on considerations of balance of interests. There are three main reasons for this. First, in order to avoid the occurrence of the phenomenon of "silent complicity." The so-called "silent complicity" refers to the phenomenon that in medical lawsuits, other physicians are usually unwilling to act as expert witnesses for the patient side and provide their expertise to give unfavorable testimony against the doctor. It is equivalent to what we often call "medical care for each other." In medical litigation in the United States, the plaintiff has the responsibility to present expert witnesses and use the opinions of expert witnesses to prove that the defendant physician should abide by the standard of conduct and that the defendant's behavior did not meet the requirements of that standard. In the case of "silent complicity," the plaintiff would lose the case because he could not provide expert witnesses to prove that the defendant physician was at fault. The application of the "state the facts" principle can resolve the plaintiff's unfavorable situation caused by the physician's "silent complicity," because as long as the plaintiff can prove the occurrence of an accident or injury and other legally established elements, they can avoid being rejected due to insufficient evidence. Second, in order to better solve the problem of medical damage that cannot be substantiated when patients receive treatment in an unconscious state. When receiving treatment, patients often fall into an unconscious state because they have to inject anesthetic injections due to their condition or the need for surgery. Under these circumstances, it was impossible for the plaintiff to know the medical actions performed by the physicians, nor was it possible to specify the physicians' negligent acts. However, if the plaintiff only makes a "general allegation" of the physician's negligence and establishes a prima facie case, the case can be handed over to the jury. If the physician cannot explain the occurrence of the injury, or the explanation is not detailed enough, he will be found guilty. There is a fault. Third, physicians are closer to the evidence than patients. One of the requirements for the "facts speak for themselves" principle is that the agent or medium causing the damage must be under the defendant's exclusive control. Medical behaviors, such as recording medical records and using medical equipment, are under the exclusive control of physicians, and patients cannot approach them at all. Moreover, after the damage occurs, the doctor has sufficient time to tamper with the evidence and destroy the evidence that is unfavorable to him. There are roughly three theories on the effect of the principle of "the facts speak for themselves" in procedural law. First, the negligent inference said that its effect was only to prevent the plaintiff from losing the lawsuit, and that the defendant did not bear a heavy burden of proof as a result. Second, the presumption of negligence says that it not only enabled the plaintiff to avoid losing the lawsuit a "directive judgment," but also made the defendant bear the burden of presenting evidence. In other words, although the burden of proof does not change, the defendant bears the burden of proof for negligence, but must provide a reasonable explanation for the fact (counter-evidence) that damage may have occurred without negligence. Third, the shift in the burden of proof says that the effect is that the burden of proof has changed, and the defendant should bear the burden of proof that he was not at fault (this proof); otherwise, it is inevitable that the lawsuit will be lost.

The principle of "explain yourself with facts" in English and American legal doctrine is founded on various elements, including two, three, and four elements. Among these, the three-element approach is generally more accepted. Section 328 (D) of the Second Review of the US Tort Law, which was completed in April 1986, stipulates that there are three elements for establishing the "facts explain oneself" principle: first, the incident must be something that would not normally have happened if there was no fault; second, all other causes of responsibility, including the plaintiff and third parties, must have been fully ruled out by the evidence; third, factual negligence occurred within the scope of the defendant's obligations to the plaintiff. Only when these three elements are present at the same time can this principle be formed and applied to specific cases in judicial practice.

If the injury suffered by the plaintiff is a complication that may occur during ordinary medical treatment, the inference of the "facts speak for themselves" principle cannot be applied. For example, male reproduction after ligation, dental damage due to endotracheal intubation, and perianal swelling during enema in people with a history of perianal disease. These complications cannot be avoided during routine medical treatment, so the principle of "explain yourself with the facts" does not apply. However, in some cases, the hospital's fault is so obvious that no expert testimony is required. General common sense and experience can be used to judge, and the court can simply apply the principle of "explain yourself with the facts." For example, the gauze was left in the abdominal cavity; surgery was supposed to be performed on the affected side, but it was performed on the healthy side; even healthy organs were removed, etc.

The application of the principle of "the facts speak for themselves" does not mean that the plaintiff will definitely obtain a winning judgment. It only allows the plaintiff to establish a prima facie case in the absence of direct evidence and submit the case to the jury for decision, avoiding the risk of the case being lost or dismissed due to insufficient evidence. Because it is easier for the defendant to explain how the damage occurred, the plaintiff will be able to obtain instructions to win the case unless the defendant can provide reasonable evidence to refute the presumption of fault. If the plaintiff has established a prima facie case based on the "state the facts themselves" principle, the defendant bears the burden of presenting a satisfactory statement; otherwise, the jury will be required to judge against the defendant.

2. Germany

German law's rules on allocating the burden of proof with respect to medical damage are called "factual proof" and are mainly used to resolve cases when it is difficult for patients to prove medical intent or negligence. "Factual proof" means abstractly extrapolating the essential facts of some kind of negligence from the objective facts of harm, based on highly probable empirical rules. In this case, if the above abstract and unspecified presumptions are to be reversed and the plausibility of the presumption raised into question, the other party must prove the existence of sufficient, specific, and specific "special things" to preclude the application of the rule of thumb. "Factual proof" is a method of proof that presumes the existence of main facts based on a single indirect fact and is based on a highly probable rule of thumb.

The main content of "factual proof" is that if "a certain reason is expressed in the rules of life experience and usually evolves in a certain direction," that is, when it is considered a "stereotyped event," the existence of a "fault" element or a "causal relationship" element can be directly presumed. "Exemplary proof" uses a highly probable rule of thumb: the standard "damage would not have occurred through the defendant's fault," leaving many victims without redress. Therefore, in German practice, an atypical and less obvious rule of thumb has begun to be used as a standard of judgment. On the grounds of "the possibility of only a specific clue," it is acknowledged that it is possible to decide whether to apply "factual proof" based on the special state of each case. This is called "individual apparent proof." "Appearance proof" is a system formed through the accumulation of precedents and doctrines. It is not the same as the legal presumption expressly stipulated in substantive law. Its function is to increase the judge's free mental evidence and enable the judge to make decisions with the help of empirical rules. The facts to be proved disputed between the parties shall be judged.

In Germany's medical infringement lawsuits, only gross medical negligence is subject to a shift in the burden of proof, similar to the reversal of the burden of proof in China's current medical infringement lawsuits. Shifting the burden of proof refers to measures taken by law to reduce the burden on compensation rights holders and mitigate the unfairness caused by the principle of allocating the burden of proof. According to the principle of burden of proof allocation, it will be determined that those who should have borne the burden of proof will change their positions with each other, so as to change the ownership of the burden of proof. The shift in the burden of proof is an exception to the principle of allocating the burden of proof.

In German practice, in order to apply this shift in the burden of proof, two conditions must be met: First, it must be gross medical negligence. Major diagnostic and treatment negligence should be based on an obvious violation of the norms recognized by the medical community. Whether the physician's negligent behavior is gross negligence in diagnosis and treatment should be determined on the basis of the medical standards at the time the medical act was performed. The burden of proof of such serious medical negligence shall be on the patient requesting damage. Second, negligence in diagnosis and treatment must have a sufficient possibility of causing damage, and it is not conditional on there being a certainty between the two. Whether negligence in diagnosis and treatment is sufficient to cause damage, the judge can only judge based on the expert's medical opinions and experience; only on the basis of a medical opinion. Only when it is seen that the negligence in diagnosis and treatment has sufficient potential to cause the harm caused can it be considered that the injury satisfies this requirement.

According to the switch of the burden of proof, the infringer bears the burden of proof and should prove that there is no fault and causal relationship, while the victim requesting compensation for damages does not have to be responsible for proving the contrary facts. According to the spirit of allocating the burden of proof, if the party that bears this evidence is unable to prove, the court will order them to bear adverse legal consequences; if the party that bears this evidence succeeds in proving, unless the other party proves the opposite fact, the court shall decide that the party to this evidence wins the case. The German Federal Supreme Court often uses the method of shifting the burden of proof for persons carrying out specialized occupations when carrying out their business in violation of a certain obligation, so that the perpetrator bears the burden of proof on the fact that there was no intentional negligence in their actions and the fact that there is no causal relationship between the act and the damage. With regard to medical personnel performing medical work harming patients, there are many cases where medical personnel have made a major mistake in their treatment behavior and caused significant damage to the patient's body; it is up to the perpetrator to prove that the wrongful act was not intentionally negligent and that there is no causal relationship between the act and the damage. The main reason for this is that medical personnel are deliberately negligent, and the causal relationship is unclear due to medical misconduct, so medical personnel should bear the burden of proof in this situation where the facts are unknown.

In Germany, a theory of "obstruction of proof" also applies to medical damages actions. The so-called "obstruction of proof" generally means that when a person who does not bear the burden of proof violates the relevant obligation because of his intention or negligence in violating the relevant obligation, the party that was originally responsible for proof is unable to obtain the evidence that needs to be provided, in terms of factual determination, makes a favorable judgment on the obstructed party's claims. "Obstruction proof is mainly used to deal with new types of litigation that are highly specialized and technical, and to solve the unreasonable phenomenon of unequal litigation weapons between parties caused by the fact that only the injurer has specialized knowledge."

3. Japan

"Presumed presumption" is that in Japanese civil law theory, the principle of preliminary presumption of negligence is applied to damage compensation cases. If, according to normal circumstances, there is a "if no fault, no damage has occurred," if the plaintiff proves the occurrence of damage and the existence of general circumstances, there is a preliminary presumption that the defendant was at fault, and the defendant must prove against the fact that he was not at fault or that his actions were not at fault; otherwise, it is inevitable that the lawsuit will be lost. For example, when someone goes to the hospital to inject medicine, the patient is deaf because the doctor mistakenly injected drug A into the patient as a type B drug that should be injected into the patient. In court proceedings, the plaintiff only needs to prove that he is deaf and that he would not have been deaf had the doctor not mistakenly injected the drug. In this case, the judge will assume that the doctor is at fault, and if the doctor cannot prove that there was no wrong injection, or that the wrong injection was caused by other causes not attributable to himself, he will bear the consequences of losing the case. In Japanese medical damage compensation dispute litigation procedures, the judicial practice also relies on this principle as a guiding principle for the distribution of the burden of proof between doctors and patients.

The purpose of the "presumptive presumption" principle is to reduce the burden of proof on victims. It is mainly used to prove negligence, but also to prove the existence of a causal relationship. The position of the "presumptive presumption" principle lies between the "factual explanation of one's own fault" principle and the "factual proof" theory. In terms of its effectiveness, it is close to the theory of "apparent proof." Still, in terms of the object of the presumption, it is closer to the principle of "facts explain themselves. Since the "presumption of presumption" principle established by the Japanese practical community is mostly applied to the determination of negligence and less to presuming the causal relationship between the act of harm and the damage caused, some people also call it the "approximate presumption of fault" principle.

Under the presumption of fault principle, the plaintiff still bears the responsibility of proving fault or the existence of a causal relationship; however, the plaintiff only needs to prove objective facts sufficient to presume intentional negligence or the existence of a causal relationship, so that it can be determined that it has fulfilled its burden of proof. This preliminary presumption of fault is a method that courts have been using to substantially reduce the plaintiff's burden of proof. In cases of highly difficult technical infringement, such as medical treatment, courts have carried out this presumption of negligence operation to reduce the burden of proof on victims. Still, it is mainly used to prove negligence. In Japanese academics, the principle of "preliminary presumption of fault" can only be factually presumed as to whether the defendant was at fault or in a causal relationship. It is not a legal presumption and therefore has not reached the level of shifting the burden of proof.

4. Taiwan region of China

Section 277 of the Civil Procedure Law of the Taiwan region of China stipulates: "Those who claim facts that are beneficial to them have the burden of proving that fact." According to this regulation, it depends on the facts claimed by the party concerned and whether it is beneficial to them. If it is beneficial to themselves, that is, the burden of proof is borne by that party, that is, the party has submitted evidence and made the civil court obtain credible evidence. It can be seen that the standard for allocating the burden of proof is determined by the fact that it is beneficial to oneself. According to the medical contract relationship between the patient and the medical staff, when medical damage occurs due to the medical personnel's negligence, if the patient requests damages based on the tort, then the burden of proof is on the medical staff to prove the elements of the infringement; if the claim for damages is not fulfilled according to the contract, the burden of proof shall be borne by the debtor and medical personnel as to the fact that the cause of responsibility does not exist, that is, the fact that there is no fault. Therefore, it is more beneficial for the patient to request damages based on the legal relationship due to the non-fulfillment of the contract. Therefore, in the Taiwan region of China, in the event of a lawsuit for damages due to negligence in diagnosis and treatment, if the patient or his family claims infringement, then the burden of proof is on the victim to seek medical advice at the physician's fault.

To measure the ability of physicians and patients to prove, since the relevant medical knowledge and skills are not well known to the general public, it is really difficult to require victims to bear the burden of proof for diagnosis and treatment performed independently by physicians. In practice, in order to ease the burden of proof on victims and achieve social fairness and justice, the presumption of negligence is often used as the theoretical basis for the diagnosis and treatment of negligence. Further, in accordance with the specific circumstances of each incident, the state of interests between doctors and patients should be considered, the causes of the two parties involved in grasping the facts, the possibility of proximity, controllability of specific risks, and difficulties in going back to the incident, and the burden of proof of the parties concerned should be adjusted or transferred appropriately."

IV. Points for Assessing the Allocation of the Burden of Proof in Medical Damage in Mainland China

1. The plaintiff shall first prove negligence in general diagnosis and treatment

From the above analysis, it can be seen that each jurisdiction has different regulations on the allocation of the burden of proof for medical damage. Still, Germany, the United States, and Japan do not stipulate a complete reversal of the burden of proof in medical damage compensation disputes, but instead decide on the allocation of the burden of proof according to the circumstances of the specific case. This point is worth pondering. At the same time, there are differences between determining causal relationships and determining fault. However, generally speaking, they are all regulations on further protecting patients' rights and interests, balancing doctor-patient interests, and establishing a harmonious doctor-patient relationship. According to specific analysis, in German medical injury lawsuits, only when there is serious medical negligence in medical treatment can the hospital bear the proof of a causal relationship. On the other hand, in general, the basic rules of civil litigation still apply to the act of diagnosis and treatment of negligence, that is, the "who claims, who gives evidence" method. At the same time, serious negligence in diagnosis and treatment in Germany must be proved by the patient. This type of diagnosis and treatment may have led to damaged results or the existence of harmful results, yet the medical authorities need to bear the burden of proof that even if they are not at fault, the damage will also occur; otherwise, they will have to bear the consequences of losing the lawsuit. It can be seen from this that Germany's sharing of the burden of proof for causal relationships in medical lawsuits caused by major medical litigation negligence has changed the problem, making it difficult for plaintiffs to prove in medical lawsuits to a certain extent. While guaranteeing the rights of vulnerable patients to litigation, it also considers how to balance the interests of patients and the medical industry, which has a good reference effect on China in establishing a reasonable burden of proof in medical lawsuits.

2. The plaintiff's proof only needs to prove the existence of objective facts that are "presumably presumed" to be established

The most common application of laws in Japan and the Taiwan region of China in the burden of proof in dealing with medical damage is for the patient to prove that the physician was at fault. Under the presumption of negligence principle, the plaintiff bears the responsibility to prove that the infringement's establishment elements include negligence and the existence of a causal relationship. However, the plaintiff only needs to prove objective facts sufficient to presume intentional negligence or the existence of a causal relationship to determine that it has fulfilled its burden of proof. This is very meaningful in reducing the burden of proof on the victim and is worth learning from.

3. Changing the medical doctor's "double burden of proof" to "choose one burden of proof"

The Supreme People's Court's Certain Provisions on Evidence in Civil Litigation stipulate that in infringement lawsuits arising from medical acts, the medical side bears the burden of proof that there is no causal relationship between the medical act and the damage results and that there is no medical fault. The essence of this is to presume that the medical side has a medical fault and that there is a causal relationship, thus requiring the medical side to bear the double burden of proof: it is necessary not only to prove that there is no fault, but also to prove that there is no causal relationship. If the medical authority is unable to fully prove the above two points at the same time, it is determined that the medical authority constitutes infringement and shall bear civil liability.

The provisions of this judicial interpretation are in fact clearly in conflict with the traditional theory of infringement. Traditional infringement theory uses causal relationships as a constitutive element. When the medical side can prove that there is no causal relationship, the medical side does not constitute infringement. However, if medical authorities cannot prove that they are not at fault, they still have to bear responsibility, thus conflicting with traditional infringement theories. I have no objection to the reversal of the burden of proof for medical disputes in China's judicial practice, but the current "double burden of proof" rule for medical doctors is indeed flawed. When issuing a judicial interpretation on the application of the Tort Liability Law, the Supreme People's Court should clearly state that in medical damage compensation cases, it is first necessary to prove "no-fault." If the medical side can prove that "there is no fault," then it is not necessary to prove that "there is no cause and effect," the court can be found exempt from liability; if the medical side cannot prove "no longer at fault," the court can be found exempt from liability. The bank requires the doctor to prove that "there is no causal relationship."

Asking physicians to prove "no causal relationship" without exception is actually unscientific. The reason is that the ability to prove causality is closely related to the degree of human mastery of science and technology and the degree of human understanding of the laws of nature. Especially in the medical field, the physiology and pathological mechanisms of the human body are extremely complex, and there are also large individual differences in the human body. There are still many unrecognized fields of medicine. Knowledge about many diseases is still very limited, and the treatment results for many diseases are not satisfactory. On the one hand, many medical problems still need to be explained by experience, which can not reach the level of "proof" completely relying on objective evidence. On the other hand, the causes of diseases are complex, not "either or," and there is often a phenomenon of "multiple causes and one result." Its causal relationship cannot be completely identified by "complete" or "none." How do we assess the phenomenon of several causes of injury acting together to cause one type of damage? Who is the main reason? Who is the secondary reason? If all of these are required for hospitals to find evidence to prove them one by one, the difficulties involved are obvious. For example, the Hubei Longfeng fetal compensation case was a sensation all over the country. The key to the hospital's failure in this case is the rule that reverses the burden of proof. The medical side suffered an unfavorable outcome of the lawsuit because it was unable to prove that there was no causal relationship. The plaintiff argued that it was the power failure of the thermostat that caused the children to get cold, suffocate, and lack oxygen, which ultimately caused the two children to have cerebral palsy. The defendant did not deny the fact that the heater was out of power, but suggested that children with cerebral palsy were generally due to congenital genetic factors, and that cold was not the main cause. Since the burden of proof was reversed, the court required the medical doctor to prove this statement. However, the causes of many diseases are still unclear, and the causes of some diseases, such as cerebral palsy, are still only hypothetical. As a result, the hospital was unable to prove causation and lost the case.

4. Legal exemption from defendant's burden of proof

The Medical Malpractice Handling Regulations stipulate six situations that are not medical malpractice. This has become an exemption and defense matter in medical malpractice litigation practice. However, since the Medical Malpractice Handling Regulations are only administrative regulations, courts can often only "refer" to the above exemptions and defense matters in judicial practice. Once the statutory exemptions defined in the General Provisions of the Tort Liability Law and Chapter 7 Medical Damage Liability are met, the defendant should be exempted from the burden of proof. However, the defendant should fulfill the burden of proof for statutory exemptions and defense matters.

Identification Rights of Medical Accidents

The identification of medical accidents is the technical identification and examination of medical accidents. Through investigation and research, it judges the nature of the disputes, analyzes the reasons for the disputes, points out the relationship between the causes and the results, and clarifies the main responsible person and other responsible persons based on the facts and guided by medical science. The right to identification is a key issue in the theory and practice of identification. The traditional view is that the right of identification is the dominant power within the scope of the duty of identification. In the author's opinion, the right to identify medical accidents can only be regarded as a state power in general, which is the dominant force in the exercise of the duty of identification. It regulates and restricts all the activities of the subject of power within the scope of duties of identification, such as the initiation and implementation of identification, the division of authority of the identification department, and the legal norms of identification practices. At the same time, depending on the identification right in different stages of medical accident handling and its connotation, it is controlled and exercised by different organs and individuals. Based on this, identification rights can be classified into five aspects: starting rights, organization rights, implementation rights, management rights, and legislation rights.

I. Starting Rights

The starting right of identification refers to the power of the administrative and judicial departments with identification rights under laws and administrative regulations or the right of the parties to initiate activities to identify medical accidents. The starting right of identification is the legal prerequisite for the right of identification to be put into practice and is also the legal basis for entrusting identification. The power to decide whether to carry out identification activities based on the decision of the authority provided for by law can also be called the decision-making power of identification. It can be argued that the starting right of identification encompasses the decision-making power of identification. Both initiate identification activities on their own initiative, but the decision-making power of identification specifically refers to the public power that can initiate identification activities.

The Regulation on the Handling of Medical Accidents (hereinafter referred to as the Regulation) firstly clarifies the starting right of identification in Chapter III, "Technical Identification of Medical Accidents." The Regulation specifies, in Article 20, three circumstances in which the identification of medical accidents may be initiated:

(1) Where the administrative department of health receives the report of any medical institution about any serious negligent medical acts and finds it necessary to make a technical identification of the medical accident, it shall have the identification done by the societies of medical sciences that are in charge of authenticating medical accidents technologically.

(2) Where the administrative department of health receives the application of the party to any medical dispute for handling and finds it necessary to make a technical identification of the medical accident, it shall have the identification done by the societies of medical sciences that are in charge of authenticating medical accidents technologically.

Where both the physician and the patient agree to settle the medical dispute through mediation and a technical identification for the medical accident is needed, the identification shall be made by the society of medical sciences in charge of technical identification upon the joint entrustment of both parties.

The first two circumstances are the transfer of the identification by the health administrative department, falling within the decision-making power of identification in the starting right of identification. In 1987, the State Council promulgated and implemented the Measures for the Handling of Medical Accidents (hereinafter referred to as the Measures). The Measures stipulate that patients, their families, and healthcare institutions may request the local technical identification committee of medical accidents for identification in case of any dispute over the confirmation or treatment of a medical incident or accident. In case of dissatisfaction with the conclusions of the Technical Identification Committee of Medical Accidents, the patient, his/her family, and the medical institution may apply for re-identification to a higher level of the Technical Identification Committee of Medical Accidents within 15 days from receipt of the conclusions. Accordingly, the subject who requests technical identification of medical accidents may be the patient and his/her family members or the medical institution. The health administrative department only bases its administrative treatment on the final and uncontested identification conclusions. It can be seen that the starting right of identification is in the hands of the parties involved in the resolution of medical accidents by the health administrative department. However, the health administrative department is generally placed in a passive waiting position.

The Regulation changes the health administrative department from waiting passively for the handling of medical accidents to intervening in advance with appropriate initiative. That is to say, under certain conditions, the health administrative department shall have the right to entrust the corresponding societies of medical sciences with the task of organizing the technical identification of medical accidents and actively monitoring the quality of medical services. To some extent, the health administrative department has the public power to determine whether or not to conduct identification. While the author is worried about the enforcement of the Regulation, he must remind everyone that in implementing the Regulation, the term "medical accidents requiring technical identification" should be correctly interpreted. Some medical accidents do not need to be technically identified by experts, but they can be correctly concluded by most citizens. If such "gross medical negligence" and "medical accident disputes" are transferred for technical identification of medical accidents, it has no practical significance but rather increases the financial burden of both doctors and patients. Moreover, it runs counter to the principle of timely and convenient handling of medical accidents. In deciding whether it is "neces-sary" or "not necessary" to perform the technical identification of medical accidents, the administrative department of health should take the ability to determine whether it is a medical accident or not as the only criterion. The technical identification of medical accidents is highly specialized, tech-nically sophisticated, and complex. In this regard, the health administrative department should act cautiously and within the limits of its means when making a judgment. The administrative department of health may decide on its own whether or not a case is a medical accident if the facts are clarified, the circumstances are simple, the dispute is minor, and it does not involve the determination of the degree of disability and the extent of the liability of the medical action in the consequences of the medical damage. In addition, the identification of medical accidents should be transferred to the societies of medical sciences, which are responsible for the technical identification of medical accidents. Otherwise, there is a high risk that the patient may file an administrative review or administrative lawsuit.

The Regulation specifies the third circumstance in which the identifi-cation of medical accidents can be initiated, whereby the identification is jointly commissioned by both the doctor and the patient. In this case, both the doctor and the patient fail to reach a consensus on the fact of medical damage incurred, its causes, the extent of damage, and the degree of liability of medical negligence in the consequences of the damage. However, both parties agree to negotiate on the basis of technical identification of the med-ical accidents to resolve the above dispute. It is clear that the starting right of identification is in the hands of the parties. At this point, the starting right of identification must also meet the following three conditions: (1) The doctor and the patient should jointly apply technical identification of medical ac-cidents. (2) The doctor and the patient should provide the medical records and physical objects needed for identification at the request of the identifi-cation agency. (3) They should accept the investigation of the identification agency and truthfully present the relevant materials.

When medical accidents are resolved through judicial means, the start-ing right of identification has changed. In China's litigation law, different provisions can be found on the initiation of identification. Article 72 of the Civil Procedure Law states, "When a people's court deems it necessary to make an evaluation of a specialized issue, it shall refer the issue to an authentication department authorized by law for the evaluation. In the absence of such department, the people's court shall appoint an authentication department to make the evaluation." Similar provisions are stipulated in Article 35 of the Administrative Procedure Law. It can be seen that the Civil Procedure Law and the Administrative Procedure Law confer the starting right of identification on the people's courts. Article 119 of the Criminal Procedure Law states, "When certain special problems relating to a case need to be solved in order to clarify the circumstances of the case, experts shall be assigned or invited to give their evaluations." However, there is no explicit provision stipulating who has the right to "assign or invite experts to give their evaluations." In practice, it is mostly the public security, procuratorate, and court departments.

Clearly, the starting right of judicial identification of medical accidents in China is vested in the hands of the courts, the procuratorates, and the public security departments to a large extent. The provisions of the Criminal Procedure Law only state that the parties and their defenders and agents ad litem have the right to apply for identification. However, the application for identification is not the hiring of identification, nor is it the decision on identification. The final decision rests with the court, which "shall decide whether or not to approve the application." The final decision rests with the court, which "shall decide whether or not to approve the application." If the court rejects the application, the person concerned can only submit to it. He or she cannot hire an appraiser and request the court to summon him or her, nor can he or she raise any query or apply for judicial relief to other relevant authorities. If, due to the omission of the people's court, the accident subject to identification is not identified, the rights of the party concerned will be infringed upon.

In common law countries, in response to adversarial litigation systems, identification procedures are generally initiated directly by the prosecutor and the defender, either by the parties or their statutory agents. Prosecutors and defense attorneys can directly commission expert witnesses to conduct identification. On the contrary, civil law countries mostly adopt ex officio litigation procedures. Identification is regarded as an activity that "helps the adjudicator to discover the truth and realize justice." Therefore, judicial identification is generally decided by the judge at the request of the parties or at his own initiative on the basis of his authority. China's identification system has a strong tone of ex officio doctrine, with the shortcomings caused by the lack of constraints on the opposing sides. The conclusion of identification is often drawn by one person, which is likely to lead to the biased belief of the judges. The common law countries implement a system in which both the prosecutor and the defender decide on the matters of identification. Because of the constraints of the opposing sides, it can usually reveal the facts of the case more comprehensively and is conducive to the trial judge hearing both parties. However, because the expert is invited by the parties, the expert may unconsciously be inclined when choosing materials for identification and drawing a conclusion.

The defense system for court trials of the common-law system has been introduced into China's current litigation system (Article 160 of the Criminal Procedure Law provides that "With the permission of the presiding judge, the public prosecutor, the parties, the defenders and the agents ad litem may state their views on the evidence and the case, and they may debate with each other."). This being the case, the parties should be granted a greater starting right of identification. As the reform of China's trial system deepens, the number of identifications initiated by the parties themselves will increase. As identification agencies are removed from their affiliation with public security agencies, prosecutors, and the courts, it is only logical that the parties should be granted the right to commission identification. From the legal point of view, the parties to medical accidents, as the most direct stakeholders in the dispute, should be the most entitled to initiate identification directly. At the same time, China is a civil law country. Concerning the judicial tradition, the starting rights of identification of the people's court and the procuratorate can not be deprived of and should co-exist with those of the parties. Still, the former should play an auxiliary role.

II. Organization Rights

The organization right of identification refers to the right of identification institutions established according to law to accept the commission of identification with corresponding qualifications and manage and coordinate the persons for identification. It is the legal basis for the establishment of identification organizations and the acceptance of identification.

The right to organize the identification of medical accidents is vested in the legal identification institutions of medical accidents. According to the latest provisions of the Regulation, there are two types of identification institutions for medical accidents: the societies of medical sciences and the institutions of judicial identification. The two types of organizations should be regarded as having the right to organize the identification of medical accidents. The societies of medical sciences are organizations for the technical identification of medical accidents organized under the administrative regulations of the State Council and confirmed by the people's governments at the same level. Their conclusions are the basis for the handling of medical accidents by administrative agencies and the judiciary.

In resolving medical accidents, forensic identification organizations attached to public security organs, procuratorates, courts, and judicial administrative organs may be entrusted if they are qualified to do so. They conduct forensic identification of the causes of medical accidents, the adverse consequences caused to the patient, and the causal relationship between the two. Their conclusions provide scientific evidence for the judicial organs in handling cases. Judicial practice has shown that the administrative departments and the former identification committees of medical accidents are increasingly overwhelmed by the task of identifying medical accidents. On the contrary, forensic agencies are playing an increasingly important role in handling medical accidents. Specifically, (1) many administrative departments are unable to deal with medical accidents and have to resort to the courts. The courts, after accepting the cases of medical accidents, seldom adopt the identification conclusions of the identification committees but instead conduct judicial identification. (2) Some medical accidents are not subject to administrative mediation but are directly brought to the courts, and the courts entrust the judicial identification.

Compared with the Measures, one of the important reforms of the Regulation is the system reform and mechanism of technical identification of medical accidents. The Measures provide for the establishment of a technical identification committee for medical accidents by administrative district in the system of identification of medical accidents. The members of the identification committee are nominated by the health administrative department and approved by the people's government of the same level. The office is located in the administrative department of health. The staff of the administrative department of health concurrently supervises the day-to-day affairs of the technical identification committee for medical accidents. The regulations summarize the experience of organizing technical identification of medical accidents in different parts of the country over the years. Combined with the characteristics, nature, and functions of technical identification of medical accidents, it is based on the principle of maximizing the scientificity and impartiality of technical identification of medical accidents. The system of the technical identification committee for medical accidents has been reformed and developed into the current system of the pool of experts for technical identification of medical accidents. In addition, the affairs of the technical identification committee for medical accidents, which was formerly undertaken by the health administrative department, were transferred to the societies of medical sciences, which are responsible for the technical identification of medical accidents.

The society of medical sciences is an independent legal person of medical and professional societies, which has no inevitable connection or interest with any organ or organization in terms of management, economy, or responsibility. It embodies the professional and intermediary nature of technical identification of medical accidents. It has changed from an identification committee to a pool of identification experts and from an administrative department of health to the societies of medical sciences. It does not represent a simple change of name or relocation of offices, but rather a major organizational and institutional change in the technical identification of medical accidents. The most prominent difference between the pool of identification experts and the identification committee is the establishment of a pool of identification experts through the societies of medical sciences, which removes the administrative element of the former identification committee from the institution. It is no longer nominated by government departments and approved by the government. The identification organization, which operates within the government department, "not administrative but also administrative," has become a unique, independent, and intermediary organization of technical identification for medical sciences. On the other hand, the expert pool is a large think-tank and reserve of high-level experts in medicine and related disciplines. It is no longer organized by a few fixed members. The members of the identification group are selected at random and are uncertain. As a result, it can better ensure that the technical identification procedures for medical accidents are open, fair, and impartial.

The author would also like to remind us that there is no hierarchy in identification. Some people think that there is a hierarchy in identification and that subordinates should obey superiors. Moreover, they hold that if there is any contradiction between the conclusion of the superior and that of the subordinate, then the conclusion of the superior should prevail. It is also a huge misunderstanding of the nature of identification. As for the identification conclusions, they are only distinguished between right and wrong, between scientific and unscientific, and there is no distinction between superior and inferior. The author has observed multiple instances where identification conclusions were made by both higher-level and lower-level identification organizations. However, it finally proves that the conclusion of the lower-level identification organization is correct. It can be seen that the validity of the identification conclusion does not come from the rank and status of the organization where the appraiser is located, but from the scientific nature of the identification process and the objective correctness of the identification conclusion.

III. Implementation Rights

The implementation right of identification refers to the right of individuals who are entitled to the right of identification in accordance with the law to perform identification of medical incidents. Specialized problems in specific cases have to be solved by means of identification. It must be realized through a series of recognition activities by appraisers with relevant expertise, i.e., identification. Article 24 of the Regulation stipulates, "The technical identification of medical accidents shall be carried out by expert identification groups organized by the societies of medical sciences responsible for organizing the technical identification of medical accidents." It indicates that technical identification of medical accidents is characterized by three features: (1) Technical identification of medical accidents must be carried out in the form of an expert identification group. (2) The expert identification group is the subject of technical identification of medical accidents. The identification expert pool is not the main body of identification, nor are the societies of medical sciences the main body of identification. The members of the expert pool are not qualified to perform identification independently without being admitted to the specialized expert identification group. (3) The expert identification group carries out identification under the organization of the societies of medical sciences that are responsible for organizing the technical identification of medical accidents.

Article 25 of the Regulation also makes it clear that the system of identification of medical accidents is collective and collegial, not a system of individual identification of experts. According to litigation science, technical identification should be the act of experts participating in litigation activities and providing expert testimony in their personal capacity. Issuing identification conclusions in the name of the identification committee formally avoids the legal responsibilities and obligations of the participants in the identification. At the same time, it deprives the identified party of the right to object and pursue the person liable for perjury.

Identification is the determination of objective facts and is a legal scientific research activity. There is only the distinction between right and wrong in science, and there is no such thing as majority rule. The purpose of the collective identification system is to eliminate the distortion caused by individual tendencies that are usually present in individual identification. However, relying on collective identification to preclude distortions caused by individual tendencies requires more stringent safeguards than individual identification. Each member of the identification committee should be able to maintain active and independent judgment and expression of opinions and be free from the influence of personal feelings, interests, and other non-technical factors. The Regulation stipulates that "where the identification of the cause of death or disability grade is involved, the forensic pathologist shall be randomly selected from a pool of experts to be a member of the expert identification group." However, under the system of collective identification, the forensic pathologist's opinion is usually excluded as a minority opinion.

At the litigation stage, the public security organs, procuratorates, and courts are the departments of the State that are entitled by law to the power of identification. For better compatibility with its functions, the implementation right of identification should be reasonably distributed depending on the functions of investigation, legal supervision, adjudication, and judicial administration. This not only ensures the relative centralization and unification of the identification right, but also facilitates the identification activities of various departments to be conducted promptly and effectively. When medical accidents are resolved through judicial identification in China, the public security organs, procuratorial organs, people's courts, and judicial administrative organs at all levels have the authority to carry out identification and have the right to organize and establish identification agencies. At the same time, they can also authorize the establishment of identification intermediary service agencies in the scientific research departments, colleges, and universities to which they belong. Whether a person or a scientific research institution has the right of identification in litigation activities, in essence, indicates whether there is the right to perform identification, and it does not imply the overall power of identification.

IV. Management Rights

The management right of identification refers to the power of administrative organization and management related to the identification of medical accidents. It guarantees the public authority for the smooth progress of identification activities. Its main components should be divided into the right to approve identification agencies, the right to grant persons for identification, the macro-guidance and regulation right of identification organizations and persons for identification, the right to coordinate, arbitrate, and supervise identification, and the right to organize scientific research for identification.

The right to approve identification agencies mainly refers to the right to appraise and review the establishment of identification agencies and to define their scale and size, establishment level, and approval procedures. The right to grant persons for identification qualification refers to the right to specifically manage and assess persons for identification, to determine the conditions and status they should have, and the procedure to obtain the qualification. The macro-guidance and regulation right of identification organizations and persons for identification means the right to examine the working status and effectiveness of identification departments at all levels and the actual working capabilities of persons for identification, and the right to decide on the promotion, rewards, and punishments of persons for identification. The right to coordinate, arbitrate, and supervise identification mainly refers to the right to coordinate and arbitrate differences in identification among departments and to supervise and manage identification agencies and personnel.

China's current system of identification of medical accidents is mainly based on departmental management. In the author's opinion, the main content of the management right is embodied in an administrative right. In addition to the health department, such an administrative right is exercised by the departments responsible for investigation, trial, and legal supervision. On the one hand, it is not conducive to better serving the judiciary through identification; on the other hand, it weakens the effectiveness and authority of the administration. For this reason, such administration should be exercised primarily by the administrative departments of the judiciary, as is the case with the administration of lawyers.

Before the reform of China's medical system is completed, in view of the continuing relationship of interest between the competent administrative department of health and hospitals, it is necessary to eliminate the undesirable effects of the current mechanism of technical identification of medical accidents in order to ensure the normal operation of the identification mechanism and the objectivity and fairness of the results of the identification. The Regulation's amendment to the Measures realizes the separation of the macro-management right of technical identification of medical accidents from the right of technical identification. That is to say, the competent health administrative department exercises the macro-management right and guidance right, and no longer specifically organizes and participates in the technical identification of medical accidents. The societies of medical sciences independently organize the technical identification. The key to the implementation of the separation of the two rights lies in whether or not the convening and organization of the meetings of the societies of medical sciences can be separated from the competent administrative department of health. Only when the societies of medical sciences are separated can the two rights be truly separated. Thus, it can ensure the independence of the societies of medical sciences and the objectivity and impartiality of the identification results.

V. Legislation Rights

The legislation right of identification means that the state organs formulate, amend, supplement, and abolish the relevant laws on the identification of medical accidents and the normative documents of identification in accordance with the scope of their duties. The legislation right of identification is one of the indispensable contents of identification rights. It is the prerequisite and basis for the creation of the right to start, organize, implement, and manage identification activities. It is also the guarantee of the power to make identification standardized and legalized.

From the source of law, China's current laws and regulations on the identification of medical accidents are, on the one hand, the provisions on identification contained in the procedural law enacted by the National People's Congress, and, on the other hand, the administrative regulations of the State Council. In terms of the origin of identification, the subject of the exercise of the legislative right of identification should also be determined in accordance with national law, specifically the National People's Congress (and its internal functional organs). Other than this, no other department or organ has the right to enact legislation on identification.

Together, the five aspects of the right to identification constitute the complete contents of the identification right. They are interrelated and inseparable. Among them, the starting right is the prerequisite for the implementation right, the management right is based on the organization right and the implementation right, and the legislative right is the foundation and basis for all rights. At the same time, these rights are essential in exercising legislative rights. Defining a clear hierarchy of the content of the right to identification is conducive to developing theoretical studies on judicial identification. Moreover, it can better guarantee the correct execution and operation of the right of identification to resolve medical accidents.

Changes and Prospects of the Emergency Treatment Agent System for Unconscious Patients

I. Significance of the Emergency Treatment Agent System for Unconscious Patients

The rule of law society should be a "free" and "autonomous" society. Generally speaking, the standard for determining freedom is—"An individual has the power to decide things on its own. One is solely responsible for acts harmful to itself."[1] The right to make independent decisions is the right to decide one's own affairs. The patient's right to make independent decisions generally refers to their right to decide their own affairs. The focus of this article is only to analyze the right to choose treatment measures in emergency treatment. The patient himself is clearly aware. Of course, the patient's opinion should be sought, but once the patient is unaware and is in emergency treatment, the law should consider establishing a complete agency system. Starting from the patient's best interests, the agent exercises the right to make autonomous decisions, so as to be as close to the patient's true wishes as possible.

---

1   Shigeru Matsui, "On the Right to Self-Determination," *Foreign Law Review*, no. 3 (1996): 11–22.

It is commonly believed that the "favorable principle" should be the primary principle of the emergency treatment surrogate system for patients who are unaware. However, as people's ideas about the quality of life, quality of death, and what is "beneficial" in favorable principles have naturally become the focus of debate, we should replace it with the "principle of respect," that is, we should try to act as an agent that is as close to the patient's true wishes as much as possible, even though this kind of behavior may not be the most beneficial to the patient in the eyes of others. This article hopes to leave aside the question of choosing treatment measures for patients who are terminally ill or have very little chance of cure, because if they are discussed with patients who want to be rescued, it can easily influence our judgment. With regard to the former, the author does not agree with the intervention of medical institutions and medical personnel, but can follow the wishes of their close relatives. Emergency treatment often does not allow sufficient time to communicate, communicate, or even preach with close relatives as normal diagnosis or elective surgery. Therefore, the law should take protecting the life safety interests of patients as the primary starting point. This is the original "patriarchal" tradition of medicine, where physicians make medical decisions in the interests of patients' lives and safety without considering the patient's wishes. Since the issue of choosing human treatment measures has historically gone from "patriarchal" physicians' decisions to modern patients' autonomous decisions, if medical institutions or medical personnel interfere with the decisions of close relatives of patients, it is easy to cause social concern, fearing that medical authorities misuse this privilege and infringe on patients' right to make autonomous decisions.

II. Changes in the Emergency Treatment Agent System for Patients with Unclear Consciousness in China

1. Era of "agents for family members, agencies, or related persons"

The Hospital Work System issued by the former Ministry of Health in 1982 included regulations on surgical signatures in its operating room work system, but it did not stipulate that patients had the right to make their own decisions. On the contrary, it stipulated that the patient's family or patient unit must sign and agree before the operation was performed. In the case of emergency surgery, if it is too late for the medical staff to obtain the consent of the family or agency, the patient's attending physician may sign and be carried out with the approval of the department director, director, or business deputy director.

Article 33 of the Regulations on the Management of Medical Institutions promulgated by the State Council in 1994 actually made some refinements and improvements based on the above provisions, dividing the decision-making power of surgery, special examinations and special treatments into three situations and stipulating them: In one case, if the patient is conscious, the patient's consent must be obtained, and the consent and signature of his family members or related persons must be obtained; in the second case, if the patient's opinion cannot be obtained, the consent and signature of his family members or related persons must be obtained; third In the three situations, if the patient's opinion cannot be obtained and there are no family members or related persons present, or other special circumstances are encountered, the attending physician shall propose a medical treatment plan and implement it after obtaining the approval of the person in charge of the medical institution or the authorized person in charge.

The author has outlined this era as an era of "agents of families or agencies, and related persons." In other words, the patient's right to make independent decisions is not established in China's laws and regulations. Instead, it requires that the consent of the patient's family or related person (such as the unit) be obtained in addition to the patient's consent. This is clearly contrary to the basic spirit of the patient's autonomy and self-determination. However, in the era of "unit people," although this provision is not satisfactory, it must also have its helplessness.

2. Era of "family agency"

In 1999, the Law on Medical Practitioners promulgated by the Standing Committee of the National People's Congress stipulated in Section 26 that physicians should truthfully explain the condition to patients or their families. Although the description of "patients or their families" is used in writing, this is the first time that China has actually established the legal status of the patient's right to make independent decisions in terms of legislation. According to the explanation of the Interpretation of the 'Medical Practitioner Law of the People's Republic of China jointly prepared by the National Office of the Legislative Affairs Committee of the Standing Committee of the National People's Congress, the former Department of Policy and Regulation of the Ministry of Health, and the former Department of Medical Administration of the Ministry of Health, in medical activities, physicians and patients are all people with independent personalities, but due to their different levels of medical knowledge, physicians have a clear difference in ability to make decisions, understand, and accept disease diagnosis and treatment. Physicians often have an active advantage. However, patients are often in a passive position. Physicians take initiative in the patient's health status and should make the best effort to relieve the patient's pain choice, but patients do not lose their independent status as a result. On the premise that treatment is not affected, physicians should respect the patient's wishes and honestly tell patients about the condition during the disease diagnosis and treatment process, so that patients can keep abreast of information on diagnosis, treatment, prognosis, etc., in a timely manner, so that they can exercise their corresponding rights to the diagnosis and treatment of the disease. Only when the patient is incapacitated or incapable of acting should the patient truthfully explain the condition to his family as an extension of the patient's ability to make independent decisions. However, legislators still have strong "good parenting" scenarios. For example, they emphasize that under the condition of the patient's informed consent, purely technical decisions should generally be based on the physician's opinion. Still, issues involving personal lifestyles and attitudes should respect the patient's wishes.[1]

The Regulations on Medical Accident Treatment promulgated by the State Council in 2002 continued the provisions of the Law on Practicing Physicians. That is, medical staff should truthfully inform patients of their condition, medical measures, medical risks, etc., and answer their inquiries in a timely manner. The emergency treatment agent for unconscious patients continues the provisions of Article 33 of the Regulations on the Management of Medical Institutions.

3. Era of "close family agency"

The provisions of Sections 55 and 56 of the Tort Liability Law in 2010 mark the evolution of China's patients' right to make independent decisions from the era of "representing the patient's family" to the era of "representing the patient's close family." First, the Tort Liability Law abolishes the use of "family members." In fact, "family" is not a strict legal term. It generally refers to family members other than yourself within the family. Its extension is vague and unclear, and in practice, it is easy to cause differences in understanding and understanding. Secondly, the Tort Liability Law chooses "close relatives" in legal terms. In commonly used legal terms, "immediate blood relatives," "side blood relatives," and "close relatives" are all used. For example, China's Marriage Law uses "immediate blood relatives" and "collateral blood relatives" within three generations. However, it is clear that the extension of "immediate blood relatives" and "collateral blood relatives" is not suitable for actual clinical use, so the Tort Liability Law finally determined that "close relatives" were used. The meaning of "close relative" differs in different legal departments in China. The "close relatives" used in civil and administrative legislation have the same meaning, and both refer to spouses, parents, children, brothers and sisters, grandparents, maternal grandparents, grand-

---

1   National People's Congress Standing Committee, Legal Affairs Committee, National Law Office, *Interpretation of the "Medical Practitioners Law of the People's Republic of China"* (Beijing: China Democratic Legal System Press, 1998).

children, and maternal grandchildren, while the scope of "close relatives" in criminal litigation legislation is smaller. It only includes husband, wife, father, mother, son, daughter, brothers and sisters. Furthermore, the Tort Liability Law and the Supreme People's Court's Interpretation on Certain Issues Concerning the Applicable Law in Trial of Medical Injury Liability Disputes (hereinafter referred to as Judicial Interpretation) both define the ranking of close relatives, and do not give priority to first-ranking close relatives to express opinions on treatment.[1]

4. No change in the status of medical institutions in the emergency treatment agent system for patients who are unaware

From the Hospital Work System to the Regulations on the Administration of Medical Institutions to the Tort Liability Law, although the "preferred agent" in the emergency treatment agent system for patients who are unaware has changed from the earliest "family member, agency, or related person" to the "family member," later "family member" to the final "close relative." However, there has never been a change in the "undercover agent" set for patient agents who are unaware of special situations in emergency treatment. The "undercover agent" referred to here means that if a patient is unconscious in emergency treatment and has special circumstances (such as poor contact with family, related persons, or close relatives), the law designates a unit or individual to act on behalf of the patient with the right to make independent decisions, with a view of making clinical decisions that are most beneficial to the patient. However, the law does not specify the formal requirements for the relevant person in charge to agree to the statement of intent. For example, the person responsible should be clearly required to sign and keep the medical record.

---

1   Shen Deyong and Du Wanhua, *Supreme People's Court Judicial Interpretation of Medical Injury Liability: Understanding and Application* (Beijing: People's Court Press, 2018), 330.

III. Regrets about the Emergency Treatment Agent System for Patients with Unclear Consciousness in the Judicial Interpretation

Although Article 33 of the Regulations on the Administration of Medical Institutions established an emergency treatment agent system for patients who are unconscious in China, the attending physician should propose a medical treatment plan, and the "other special circumstances" in which treatment is carried out after obtaining approval from the head of the medical institution or the person authorized to be responsible have not been refined. After the enactment of the Tort Liability Law, there has been an academic dispute over whether "unable to obtain the opinions of patients or their close relatives," as stipulated in Article 56, only indicates that the opinions of patients or their close relatives cannot be objectively obtained,[1] that is, the patients themselves are unable to express their intentions and cannot identify or contact their close relatives for a while, or whether they are subjectively unable to obtain the opinions of patients or their close relatives, including cases where the patient's close relatives refuse to agree or cannot reach agreement. Whether to agree "unable" includes "cases where patients or their close relatives clearly refuse to take medical measures," academics can probably be divided into "theory of approval" and "theory of opposition."

1. Theory of approval

According to the legislative explanation of the National People's Congress Legal Affairs Committee, as early as December 2008, when the Tort Liability Law (Draft) was submitted to the National People's Congress Standing Committee for second review, this provision stipulated: "In emergency situations such as rescuing dying patients, if it is difficult to obtain the consent

---

1   Chen Te, "On the Special Provisions of Medical Institutions' Duty to Notify: Discussion on Legal Issues in a Medical Injury Compensation Dispute Case between Mr. Li and Others and a Beijing Hospital," in *Frontiers of Examination and Approval: Trial Practice in New Types of Cases: Episode 34 of the Total*, ed. Beijing Higher People's Court (Beijing: Law Press, 2011), 53.

of the patient or his close relatives, corresponding medical measures can be implemented immediately with the approval of the person in charge of the medical institution." The expression "difficult" here can easily be understood to include "situations where the patient or their close relatives clearly disagree." Later, according to opinions from various parties, it was revised to "not possible," considering that although "cases where patients or their close relatives clearly disagree with treatment" do occur in practice, there is no agreement on how to handle it, and there is a lot of disagreement, so it will be clearly stipulated when conditions are ripe in the future. Therefore, it can be assumed that "unable to obtain the opinions of patients or their close relatives" refers to situations where patients cannot express their intentions, are not accompanied by close relatives, and are unable to contact close relatives, not including cases where the patient or their close relatives have clearly indicated that they refuse to take medical measures.[1]

Some scholars support this view, arguing that the Tort Liability Law legislation is intended to limit situations where opinions cannot be obtained from patients or their close relatives to objectively impossible, that is, where close relatives are unknown or have no contact information, or where contact information is available but close relatives cannot be reached. For example, the victim of a traffic accident is in a coma, has no information on his body that can prove his identity, and is unable to contact his close relatives. As for the patient being able to express his intentions and clearly refusing to agree, or if the patient is unable to express his intentions but his close family clearly refuses or does not reach an agreement, the decision of the closest relative is clearly not conducive to the patient's situation. Section 56 of the Tort Liability Law does not apply, and the patient cannot demand responsibility from the medical institution as a result. The consequences of damage caused by the patient's close relatives refusing to sign shall be borne by them in accordance with Article 60 (1) of the Tort Liability Law. There are two reasons: First, when close relatives refuse to express an opinion or cannot reach an agreement, or are still making such decisions in the knowledge that the decision is unfavorable to the patient, it is difficult to

---

1   Wang Shengming, *Explanation of the Provisions and Legislative Background of the Tort Liability Law of the People's Republic of China* (Beijing: People's Court Press, 2010), 220.

say that it is appropriate for the medical institution to intercede someone in the anchor section between the patient and the close family. This even provided an excuse for patients or their close relatives to refuse to pay the corresponding expenses later and make unreasonable excuses to demand that medical institutions assume responsibility. Second, when all of the patient's close relatives are on the scene unconcerned about the patient's life or death and are even slow to reach an agreement, patients in a coma can only admit that they are unlucky; they must bear the risk of such a bad and desperate relative on their own.[1]

2. Theory of opposition

It holds that in the triangular relationship between patients, medical institutions, and the patient's close relatives, the subjective status and decision-making power of the patient's close relatives cannot be set too high. If the opinions of patients cannot be obtained, only the opinions of their close relatives can be obtained. There should be some margin of judgment on how medical institutions take emergency treatment measures. When the opinions of patients' close relatives are significant and clearly harm the patients' interests, medical institutions should refuse to accept the opinions of close relatives of patients.[2] Yang Lixin classified it as ethical negligence. If it is believed that it is difficult to obtain the consent of the patient or their close relatives due to an emergency situation such as rescuing a critical patient, the corresponding medical measures may be implemented immediately with the approval of the head of the medical institution. Violation of the aforesaid obligation described above constitutes medical negligence. Zhang Xinbao[3] also believes that Section 10 of the Basic Code for Writing Medical Records issued by the former Ministry of Health in 2010 gave heads of medical institutions to sign and allow the execution of rescue measures to

---

1   Cheng Xiao, *Tort Liability Law*, 2nd ed. (Beijing: Law Press, 2015), 561–562.

2   Xi Xiaoming, *Understanding and Application of the Provisions of the Tort Liability Law of the People's Republic of China* (Beijing: People's Court Press, 2010), 404–405.

3   Zhang Xinbao, *Tort Liability Law*, 4th ed. (Beijing: China Renmin University Press, 2016), 222.

rescue patients when close relatives of patients are unable to sign, so as to avoid situations where emergencies that endanger the lives of patients, rescue actions that can determine the life and death of patients must be subject to helplessness by families of patients who do not understand medicine. Of course, this statement also agrees that as a treatment of the patient's own rights, it should be respected and protected by law on the premise that it does not violate mandatory law and basic social ethics.[1]

3. "Judicial Interpretation": A difficult choice between two schools of view

Article 20 of the Interpretations of the Supreme People's Court on Several Issues Concerning the Application of Law in the Trial of Medical Damage Liability Dispute Cases (hereinafter referred to as the Draft for Comments) stipulates the circumstances and legal responsibilities for emergency treatment and details the provisions: "In the following situations, when the patient is in critical condition and unable to express his opinion, with the approval of the person in charge of the medical institution or the authorized person in charge, corresponding medical measures can be implemented immediately to save the patient's life: (1) The close relatives are unknown or have no contact information. (2) There is contact information, but the close relatives cannot be contacted. (3) The close relatives refuse to express opinions. (4) The opinions of close relatives are inconsistent, and a majority opinion cannot be formed. (5) The opinions of close relatives are obviously not conducive to the patient's interests. (6) Other situations stipulated by laws and regulations. Under the circumstances of the preceding paragraph, if a medical institution and its medical staff fail to immediately implement corresponding medical measures and cause harm to the patient, and the patient requests the medical institution to bear compensation liability, the People's Court shall support it. The Draft for Comments has not yet been formally adopted and promulgated. In 2015, the Guangzhou Intermediate People's Court took the lead in learning from the provisions of Article 20 of

---

1   Elken and Qin Yongzhi, "On Medical Informed Consent: A Review of the Provisions of Sections 55 and 56 of the Tort Liability Law," *Eastern Methodology*, no. 3 (2010): 109–115.

the Draft for Comments. It made exactly the same provisions in Article 36 of the Guidelines for the Trial of Medical Damage Liability Dispute Cases promulgated by it.

However, in repeated discussions among all parties in the Draft for Solicitation of Comments, the most controversial point was that "(5) the opinions of close relatives are clearly not conducive to the interests of patients" were eventually removed. In fact, it is mainly medical representatives who oppose its inclusion in judicial interpretation because they are concerned that this regulation will be difficult to grasp in clinical practice. In view of the relevant medical laws and regulations, diagnosis and treatment regulations, and judgment based on the circumstances of the specific case, this aspect involves balanced protection of doctors' and patients' interests, as well as medical ethics issues, and should be carefully grasped. For example, for critically ill patients who cannot express their opinions, and there are situations where the opinions of close relatives cannot be obtained, this is clearly stipulated in the Medical Practitioners Law, but to what extent the treatment risk is. First of all, it is necessary to respect the professional judgment of medical institutions and carefully consider it. There is indeed a need to explore this major medical ethics issue between "good death" and "staying alive" in practice further.

The drafter also pointed out in the explanation of this underwriting clause (5) Other circumstances stipulated by law or regulation] that although there are opinions that this section does not need to specify the undercover clause, after research, it is necessary to reserve other situations stipulated in this law and regulation in consideration of the complexity of social life. This not only maintains the openness of the application of the judicial interpretation itself, but also addresses the urgency of the patient's condition. It also includes situations where it is too late to seek the opinions of the patient's close relatives in the future. How to determine situations where it is too late to solicit opinions from patients' close relatives is also a matter of professional judgment. In this regard, it is necessary to respect not only the professional judgment of medical personnel during diagnosis and treatment, but also relevant professional opinions in post-factual dispute handling.[1]

4. In three special situations, medical personnel must intervene and apply the underwriting clause of Article 18 of the Judicial Interpretation

Whether the "unable" in "unable to obtain the opinion of the patient or his close relatives" stipulated in Article 56 of the Tort Liability Law includes "situations in which the patient or his close relatives expressly refuse to take medical measures" shall depend on the specific circumstances, the author still agrees with the expression in the Draft for Comments (taking "the opinions of close relatives that are obviously not conducive to the interests of the patient" as a special situation). According to civil law theory, if a parent or guardian performs an act that is obviously detrimental to a person who lacks capacity, the civil act will be invalid. First of all, if the patient is terminally ill or has a very low chance of cure and the close relatives clearly express their refusal to take medical measures before death, medical staff should respect the wishes of the close relatives. As mentioned above, this situation does not actually fall into the category of "the opinions of close relatives are obviously detrimental to the interests of the patient" and should be eliminated first to avoid confusing the public.[2]

In the following three common situations, medical staff should not listen to the opinions of close relatives who refuse medical treatment: first, due to asymmetry in knowledge between the doctor and patient, the patient's close relatives have greatly misunderstood the contents of the medical staff's instructions and refuse to treat patients who want to be rescued; second, the patient's close relatives have no major misunderstanding about what the medical staff told them, but they have bad intentions to hurt the patient's

---

1   Guo Feng, Wu Zhaoxiang, and Chen Longye, *A Guide to the Interpretation and Practice of Supreme People's Court Judicial Interpretation Provisions on Medical Injury Liability Disputes* (Beijing: China Legal System Press, 2018).

2   Su Li, "Informed Consent and Personal Freedom and Responsibility in Health Care: From Xiao Zhijun's Visa Refusal Case," *Chinese Law*, no. 2 (2008): 3–27.

life safety; third, the patient himself commits suicide, and the close family refuses to treat patients who wish to be rescued. There are three main reasons: First, emergency clinical treatment is often short of time. If you really understand the medical situation, you will find that when medical personnel face close relatives who lack a medical background and a sufficient foundation of trust, it is difficult to achieve the "informed consent" required by law in a short period of time, allow close relatives to "fully understand," and obtain "true expressions of intent" from close relatives, so it is not surprising that close relatives have "major misunderstandings." Second, when patients or close relatives have the above three situations, medical personnel must intervene, because this is not only an "ethical issue." When patients enter a medical institution, they have formed a legal relationship rather than a social relationship with the medical institution. Third, the precondition that a civil act has a legal effect is a "true expression of intent" and is not contrary to public order and morals. Among the three situations mentioned above, the first type is a close relative's statement of intent that clearly has a major misunderstanding and is not a true statement of intent (this situation often manifests as close relatives rejecting some kind of treatment measure recommended by the medical staff, but on the other hand, at the same time requiring that the patient's life must be treated. This is very important. Many scholars confuse "refusing treatment" with "refusing treatment given by a doctor," which can easily lead to misjudgment[1]). The latter two situations are contrary to public order and morals, so medical personnel must intervene. Although scholars cite the case of Jehovah's Witnesses in the US in support of respecting the autonomy of patients or close relatives,[2] such cases cannot justify the actions of medical personnel.[3] The reason the US judge asked medical personnel to respect the patient's wishes, in this case, is because in the interests protected by law, life must give way to faith, that is, when we weigh the right to life and the right to freedom of belief, we need to be aware

---

1   Su Li, "Informed Consent and Personal Freedom and Responsibility in Health Care: From Xiao Zhijun's Visa Refusal Case," *Chinese Law*, no. 2 (2008): 3–27.

2   Ibid.

3   Zhuang Xiaoping, "Also on Informed Consent and Personal Freedom and Responsibility in Health Care: A Discussion with Professor Su Li," *Natural Dialectics Newsletter*, no. 1 (2012): 116–120.

that people with religious beliefs may abandon their lives and defend their beliefs, which rooted in the belief that life without one's faith is inferior to death. Moreover, my willingness to give up rescue because of my faith is a "statement of true meaning," which is completely different from the patient in an emergency. Due to "major misunderstandings," the "meaning is clearly disadvantageous to the patient."[1] Since "the opinions of close relatives are clearly detrimental to the interests of patients" have been removed from the "Judicial Interpretation," it is recommended to use underwriting clauses to cover this situation. Otherwise, on the surface, we have strictly complied with laws and regulations, but in essence, we are violating laws and regulations.[2]

IV. Trends and Prospects of the Emergency Treatment Agent System for Patients with Unclear Consciousness

1. From "doctor-centrism" to "patient-centrism"

Figure 2 is a schematic diagram of the three eras experienced by the emergency treatment agent system for patients who are unaware. It clearly shows the changing legislation trend on patients' right to make independent decisions in China. The author summarizes this trend as a change from "doctor-centrism" to "patient-centrism." The Hospital Work System and the Regulations on the Administration of Medical Institutions do not specify the patient's right to make independent decisions but instead stipulate that the consent and signature of the patient's family or–unit (person concerned)

---

1   Wang Yue, "On Physicians' Treatment Privileges in Emergency Medical Care: Scope of Application of Section 56 of the Tort Liability Law," *Chinese Forensic Examination*, no. 4 (2011): 50–54.

2   Shangguan Piliang, "We Should Use the Concept of Putting the Right to Life First to Understand Medical Regulations: Implications Left for Us by the 'Death of a Pregnant Woman' Incident," *Jurisprudence*, no. 12 (2007): 8–12.

must also be obtained. In addition to being related to the social and historical background at the time, this kind of legislative consideration can be called "doctor-centrism." The wider the range of agents that are in patients' best interests when the patient's awareness is unclear, the more convenient it is for doctors to work. However, starting with the "Medical Practitioners Law" in 1999, China actually established a system of independent decision-making power for patients and no longer allowed patient units (stakeholders)–to act as agents in the best interests of patients; further, in 2010, agents with the patient's best interests were reduced from family members to close relatives. It may be inconvenient to act as agents for doctors, but the narrowing of the scope of agents is undoubtedly more beneficial to surrogate opinions close to the patient's own expression, so it can be called "patient centrism."

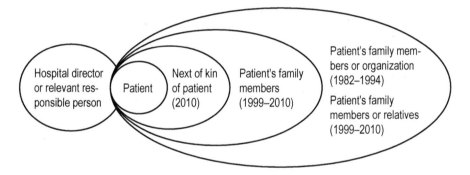

Figure 2. The three eras experienced by the emergency treatment agent system for unconscious patients

2. From "provision doctrine" to "case doctrine"

As mentioned above, although the deletion of "the opinions of close relatives are clearly detrimental to the interests of patients" is the biggest regret of Section 18 of the Judicial Interpretation," the current underwriting clause (other circumstances stipulated by laws and regulations) can also reserve room and room for maneuver for complex clinical situations in the future. Due to the complexity of the clinical situation, it is actually difficult to enumerate the specific situations of various patients through the "legal provisions." In China's emergency treatment agent system, the law should establish an "undercover agent" for the interests of patients who are unconscious under special circumstances. This agent can make final clinical decisions through individual case reviews and discussions. Currently, the "undercover agent," as stipulated in China's law, is the head or authorized person in charge of a medical institution. In clinical practice, many medical institutions have adopted internal rules and regulations to specify the performer as the head of the medical service department and the administrative duty officer. In the context of the gradual de-administration of medical institutions, legislation should be passed requiring all medical institutions to establish a "clinical ethics committee" to act as "underwriting agents."

3. From "legalism" to "intention doctrine"

The laws of some developed countries stipulate that when patients have the ability to decide, they can make specific medical predictions, medical instructions, or designated agents for treatment after losing the ability to decide on their own illness, so as to ensure that once patients lose their ability to decide, they can still be treated according to their own wishes. Furthermore, in many countries, the right to choose euthanasia is also viewed as part of the patient's right to decide for themselves. Although China's laws already establish an emergency treatment agent system for unconscious patients, this is a protective system with a backup nature, and the medical industry should vigorously promote medical predictions, medical instructions, or designated agents. Allow the patient to make his or her own advance directive or intended authorization while he or she is still aware. This is undoubtedly more humane and more humane. Some scholars have pointed out that in addition to the patient's consent, there are two special ways to exercise the right to informed consent in practice. The Tort Liability Law does not explicitly stipulate this, and future judicial interpretations should provide for it. The first type is to authorize others to exercise. The second type is to authorize medical institutions to make decisions.[1] For example, some civil society organizations in China have begun to make certain ef-

---

1   Wang Zhu, *Special Study on Difficult Issues in Tort Liability Law* (Beijing: Renmin University Press, 2012), 77–78.

forts in this regard, objectively promoting the development of Death with Dignity. For example, in May 2009, the "Choice and Dignity" public welfare website released the first folk text, "My Five Wishes," recommended for use in mainland China. By promoting "My Five Wishes," more people can understand what a "pre-life prophecy" is and how to use "pre-life prophecy" to pre-dispose the risks they may encounter when they pass away.[1]

---

1 Wang Yue, "On Death with Dignity," *Journal of Jiangsu Police Academy* 27, no. 3 (2012): 81–88.

Evolution and Prospect of Medical Negligence in China from the Perspective of Tort Law in the UK

I. Medical Negligence in British Tort Law

In British tort law, negligence and duty of care are synonymous. In the 1932 Donoghue vs. Stevenson case, the concept and principle of duty of care began to be developed. The so-called duty of care is an obligation for the perpetrator to take reasonable care to avoid damage to the person or property of others. After this case, the duty of care gradually extended from neighbors to many professionals, including physicians. Although medical negligence is part of tort law in traditional British tort law, there is now a trend of independence from tort law.[1]

1. From "Bolam test" to "Bolam/Bolitho test"

> *"Bolam test"*

The most important test of whether physicians have fulfilled their duty of care is the 1957 Bolam vs. Friern case (hereinafter the "Bolam case"). Mr. Bolam, 54, is suffering from depression. In the absence of anesthesia, the

---

1   Xu Aiguo, *Anglo-American Tort Law* (Beijing: Peking University Press, 2004), 103.

defendant gave him electroshock therapy. Although Mr. Bolam signed a consent form for treatment, he was unaware that the treatment may have a fracture risk. In the seizure-induced phase of the seizure, Mr. Bolam had a pelvic fracture. According to Mr. Bolam, the physicians did not use muscle relaxants or provide protective restraint support at the time. Medical experts appointed by the court agreed that if Mr. Bolam had been given anesthesia, the fracture would not have occurred. However, medical experts also believe that there are two common practices: one is anesthetic, and the other is non-anesthetic, and both methods were recognized by the industry at the time. In this case, Judge McNair wrote in his instructions to the jury: "The so-called test standards are the standards that practitioners who are usually proficient in a certain skill should meet. A practitioner doesn't have to have the best professional skills; the rule of law is that if the practitioner has implemented the usual skills of his peers, that's enough. Medical negligence means not meeting the qualified skills that general physicians had at the time. There may be one or more perfect and appropriate standards, but if a medical worker meets one of these appropriate standards, he should not be considered negligent. If a physician's medical behavior is acceptable to responsible peers, then he/she is not responsible. In the field of diagnosis and treatment, sufficient space should be given to accommodate different perspectives, and he/she should not be held responsible for negligence solely because his/her conclusions differ from those of other professionals.

The judge ultimately held that the doctor's behavior met the standards of a "responsible medical staff" and that the doctor did not commit medical negligence and was not responsible for the patient's hip injury. At the same time, the judge believed that medical experts who can assist in making negligence judgments should have the "3R standard," that is, responsible, reasonable, and respected.[1] After the Bolam case, the "Bolam test" was applied to all types of medical professionals' due diligence trials. For example, a physician suspects that a patient is likely to have tuberculosis but does not rule out lung cancer. The physician chose not to wait for the results of a sputum test to diagnose tuberculosis and immediately performed

---

1   Samuels A., "The Clinical Duty of Care: Is It Enough That the Doctor Did What All or Many of the Other Doctors Do?," *Med Sci Law* 46, no. 1 (2006): 76–80.

a mediastinoscopic biopsy to diagnose lung cancer, which carries the risk of complications. Assuming the patient has complications and the biopsy results are negative, the patient is eventually diagnosed with tuberculosis. Medical experts often agree with physicians' current practices when they appear in court. Then, even if the judge doesn't quite agree with the medical expert's testimony, he has to use it as the basis for finding fault. The "Bolam test" clearly benefits the medical community; that is, as long as a physician earnestly implements the practices that other physicians would take in the same situation, it is not negligent.

> ### Questions about the "Bolam test"

The "Bolam test" is performed by medical experts, and almost all experts are from the medical community. Because the "Bolam test" is physician-based, it has always been criticized by some academics, critics, and public organizations. Some argue that the use of the "Bolam test" by the courts is a dereliction of duty to protect patients' rights.[1] Often, experts stick to their role as physicians, do not "think empathically," but only make judgments based on physicians' work habits. This is why it often happens: after passing the "Bolam test," patients are unaware of the medical risks they should clearly be told about. These practices, which jeopardize patients' autonomy, are increasingly causing the judicial authorities to question the "Bolam test." However, the "Bolam test" is different from the US. Instead of using physicians' standards to conduct fault tests, US judges judge whether physicians have fulfilled their duties based on the patient's reasonable expectations.

> ### "Bolam/Bolitho test"

The most instructive challenge to the "Bolam test" is the Bolitho case. Bolitho is a 3-year-old child with asthma. There were three times of shortness of breath after admission. The first two times, an anesthesiologist came to the consultation and decided that intubation was not needed for the time being. The anesthetist did not attend when she called to inform her of the third consultation. The court found that even if she did attend, she would have

---

1 Young A., "Review: The Legal Duty of Care for Health and Other Health Disciplines," *J Clin Nurs* 18, no. 22 (2009): 3071–3078.

decided not to need intubation, just like the previous two times. In the end, Bolitho died. Judge Wilkinson ruled as follows: "The court should not be bound to find that a defendant physician can be relieved of responsibility for his negligent treatment or diagnosis simply because he has provided testimony from several medical experts who sincerely believe that the defendant's treatment or diagnosis was in accordance with proper medical practice. However, in most cases, medical experts are expected to justify their opinions. In particular, the treatments it supports are reasonable in terms of risk and benefit assessments. However, if, in rare circumstances, the court finds that the industrial views held by the defendant physician cannot withstand logical analysis and are unreasonable and irresponsible, even if there are people supporting his views, the court may find that he was negligent, even though there are supporters of his view."

The opinion of medical experts is indeed a very important piece of evidence, but it is not necessarily sufficient. When a judge reviews a medical expert's opinion, he or she may find that there is no "logical basis," such as that the corresponding risks and benefits may not have been properly weighed and assessed; there may be no reasonable reason to take this risk; medical knowledge may not be used well; Perhaps the medical knowledge used is or is becoming obsolete; it may be easier and more economical to replace it with another measure to prevent the occurrence of medical risks.[1]

Beginning with the Bolitho case, the judge began to draw a line between a finding of clinical negligence and a finding of legal negligence. Depending on the case's particular circumstances, clinical negligence may (or may not) naturally result in legal negligence. Of course, medical experts still make the relevant clinical negligence determination based on the "Bolam test." Still, the judge will use logical analysis and critical evaluation to reevaluate the medical experts' conclusions, thus creating a new standard for determining medical negligence, the "Bolam/Bolitho test."[2] Although there is no "Bolam test" that is more beneficial to doctors, the "Bolam/Bolitho test" makes

---

1 Samuels A., "The Clinical Duty of Care: Is It Enough That the Doctor Did What All or Many of the Other Doctors Do?," *Med Sci Law* 46, no. 1 (2006): 76–80.

2 Bryden D. and Storey I., "Duty of Care and Medical Negligence," *Pain Education in Anaesthetist, Critical Care & Pain* 11, no. 4 (2011): 124–127.

physicians more morally inclined to ensure that the interests of patients are maximized, which also affects and shapes their behavior. Generally speaking, physicians must resist the temptations of past habits and be willing to challenge traditional practices based on patients' best interests.

2. Medical negligence does not necessarily have reprehensible characteristics

In British tort law, the reasonable person standard is a completely objective standard of conduct. It does not use the defendant's subjective characteristics or other characteristics to determine whether the defendant's behavior is reasonable, but rather makes a judgment based on the nature of the defendant's conduct. Regardless of who the defendant is, as long as the nature of his behavior is the same, the criteria for judgment are the same; that is, the behavior of an average person in the same industry is the standard.[1] Some scholars compare his image to a "degaussing device," that is, to eliminate the defendant's subjective or personal color, and to test whether his behavior is reasonable according to the same model.[2] The consequence of this test is that not all defendants who bear liability are subjectively or morally reprehensible. Judge Denning sincerely comforted the defendant after ruling that a girl who accidentally hit and injured her instructor while a beginner driver was held responsible: "There is absolutely no need to fall into a vortex of moral self-blame for oneself."

---

1   J. Tingle, "Breach of the Duty of Care in the Tort of Conviction," *Br J Nurs* 11, no. 17 (2002): 1128–1130.

2   Hu Xuemei, *British Tort Law* (Beijing: China University of Political Science and Law Press, 2008), 119.

II. Changes in Medical Negligence in China's Legislation

1. Medical negligence as defined in the Medical Incident Handling Measures

Section 2 of the 1987 Measures for the Handling of Medical Accidents stipulated the subjective fault of the subject of the medical accident as "negligence due to diagnosis, treatment, and nursing." In 1988, the former Ministry of Health's Explanation on Certain Issues divided it into negligence and excessive self-confidence. It proposed that "acts constituting a medical accident negligence must be illegal and harmful. In a medical accident, illegality mainly refers to a violation of the rules, regulations, and technical operation procedures for diagnosis, treatment, and nursing. These can be written, or they can be conventions that everyone follows in practice." As can be seen, medical negligence as defined in the Measures for the Handling of Medical Accidents only refers to "negligence in diagnosis, treatment, and nursing," and the corresponding judgment standard is "diagnosis, treatment, and nursing standards and practices."

2. Medical negligence as defined in the Medical Malpractice Handling Ordinance

In 2002, in drafting the Regulations on the Handling of Medical Accidents, the judicial authorities pointed out that "medical treatment and nursing regulations" were insufficient to cover all medical negligence. If medical personnel did not even fulfill their general legal obligations with respect to the rights and interests of others stipulated by law, then their actions were clearly gross negligence.[1] The drafters adopted the above opinions, so they extended the criteria for judging medical negligence in medical institutions and medical personnel to "medical and health management laws, adminis-

---

[1] Tang Dehua, *Understanding and Application of the Regulations on Handling Medical Accidents* (Beijing: China Social Science Press, 2002), 37.

trative regulations, departmental regulations, and diagnosis, treatment and nursing standards and practices."

3. Medical negligence as defined in Tort Liability Law

Although there are "three elements theory" and "four elements theory" on the constitution of torts, both theories admit that fault is the essential element of torts constitution. Except for a few scholars who insist that fault is an act and an objective concept, the vast majority of scholars believe that fault, in terms of its attributes, is a subjective psychological state of a person and, therefore, a subjective concept. Of course, some scholars insist that fault is a combination of subjective and objective factors.[1] Although the mainstream view holds that fault is a subjective concept, the criteria for judging fault show an objective trend. The so-called fault standard refers to what is used to judge whether the infringer was at fault when committing the infringement. British tort law uses "the degree of care that should be achieved" as the standard for fault judgment. However, in theory, the "level of attention that should be achieved" also has a dispute between "subjective standard statement" and "objective standard statement." The "subjective standard statement" determines whether there is a fault by judging the infringer's state of mind. The "objective standard theory," which now dominates the mainstream view, is to compare the infringer's behavior through some kind of objective behavior standard, and to infer whether the infringer's subjective aspect is at fault from the external manifestations and characteristics of the infringer's behavior.[2]

After the Tort Liability Law was officially implemented in 2010, how to understand the "failure to fulfill the obligation of diagnosis and treatment corresponding to the level of medical treatment at the time" referred to in Section 57 of the Tort Liability Law is a very important issue. Wang Shengming[3] believes that fulfilling the obligation of diagnosis and treatment in-

---

1 Wang Liming, *Tort Liability Law* (Beijing: China Renmin University Press, 2016), 89.

2 Zhang Xinbao, *China's Tort Law* (Beijing: China Social Science Press, 1998), 135–136.

3 Wang Shengming, *Explanation of the Provisions and Legislative Background of the Tort Liability Law of the People's Republic of China* (Beijing: People's Court Press, 2010), 221.

cludes, of course, the requirements of laws, administrative regulations, rules, and medical standards. However, the medical staff fully complied with the above requirements, and there is still a possibility of fault. The key is to see if other health workers generally don't make this kind of mistake. A similar view also argues that medical personnel can do their part to avoid harm to patients through careful action or inaction under normal circumstances.[1] There are also opinions that the duty of care of medical personnel is the most basic obligation of medical personnel. In providing medical services to patients, medical personnel are required to exercise the best care for patients, so as to protect the lives and health of patients from harm other than the permissibility of medical treatment.[2] Some scholars believe that the duty of care of medical personnel includes the duty of care in general and the duty of special care. The former includes the obligation of all legally practicing physicians to pay attention to, while the latter includes the obligation to explain, inform, refer to a doctor, consult a doctor, observe and care, etc.[3] Other scholars believe that medical personnel are obligated to pay close attention during medical activities. The duty of high care is generally a higher duty of care than that of a good manager. Some scholars suggest that "the level of medical care at the time" is not equal to the "level of medicine at the time," and that regional factors should be taken into account. Also, "the level of medical care at the time" is not an abstract concept; it must include the two dimensions of breadth and depth. Breadth is the question of the scope of the duty of care under the medical standards at the time; depth is the question of the extent to which the duty of care must be achieved under the medical standards at the time.[4]

From a comparative legal point of view, objectification of fault judgment criteria has indeed been the development trend of tort law since the

---

1   Wang Liming, Zhou Youjun, and Gao Shengping, *Research on Difficult Issues in Tort Liability Law* (Beijing: China Legal System Press, 2012), 470.

2   Xi Xiaoming, *Understanding and Application of the Provisions of the Tort Liability Law of the People's Republic of China* (Beijing: People's Court Press, 2010), 407.

3   Gong Saihong, *Medical Injury Compensation Legislation Research* (Beijing: Law Press, 2001), 167–168.

4   Zhang Liuqing and Shan Guojun, *Summary of Adjudication of Medical Liability Disputes and Case Interpretation* (Beijing: Law Press, 2012), 188–189.

20th century, that is, starting from the need to protect victims, reducing the burden of proof on victims, making it easier for judges to judge faults, thus making the judgment of fault better serving the needs of accountability.[1] Therefore, Tort Liability Law adopts the theory of "objective standard" in fault standard. The "objective standard" is proposed as a "bonus paterfamilias" (bonus paterfamilias) standard in civil law and the "rational man" (the rational man) standard in British and American law.[2] This kind of legally designed person is not the "highest standard of conduct," nor is it a "general standard," but rather a "moderate" standard of conduct, that is, the standard of conduct for a reasonable and careful person.[3]

III. Impact and Prospects of British Tort Law on Medical Negligence in China's Judicial Practice

1. The court shall strengthen the full examination and review of medical technical assessment opinions in each case

In fact, the technical assessment of medical disputes often has problems with different expert opinions. From the Measures for the Handling of Medical Accidents to the Regulations on the Handling of Medical Accidents, the technical assessment of medical disputes follows a minority subject to a majority system, so China's standards for determining medical negligence have always been stricter than the "Bolam test."

The term "expert opinion" appeared for the first time in the Decision on the Administration of Forensic Examination, which came into effect in 2005. Section 48 of the Criminal Procedure Law implemented in 2013 also reflects a major advance in forensic examination in China—changing the

---

1   Wang Liming, *Tort Liability Law Research* (Beijing: China Renmin University Press, 2010), 330.

2   Wang Yue, *Medical Affairs Law* (Beijing: People's Health Press, 2009), 88–89.

3   Wang Liming, *Tort Law Research*, vol. 1 (Beijing: China Renmin University Press, 2004), 511.

term "forensic conclusion" stipulated in relevant laws to "expert opinion." Some scholars believe that the change from "forensic opinion" to "forensic opinion" only makes the term "expert opinion" reflect that an expert opinion is the essence of verbal evidence. Other than that, no other "statement of meaning" reduces the probative power of an appraisal opinion.[1] However, as can be seen from recent judicial practice, "forensic conclusion" to "forensic opinion" is a major shift in the concept of evidence, not a word game. The court should fully question and examine the expert opinion and decide whether to finally accept it based on the examination results and review defining opinions.

Some scholars suggest that medical malpractice assessments should not be final.[2] After the implementation of the Tort Liability Law, although the vast majority of judges found medical fault almost entirely in accordance with the medical technical assessment opinions, some judges have already begun to fully examine and examine the medical technical assessment opinions on individual cases and try to determine whether the medical technical assessment opinions have a "logical basis." The significance of this progress is very similar to the "Bolitho case." Judges have indeed tended to use the "patient-centered" standard to measure whether doctors have fulfilled their duty of care. For example, when it is necessary to determine whether physicians' information is sufficient, courts often do not speculate on medical experts' current practices; instead, they ask what rational patients would like to know in such situations. Or the judge speculates on "what the physician would wish to know if he himself were in the same situation, and what the physician would do if his friends or family members were in a similar situation."

Judges always play a difficult role in medical damages lawsuits because they must balance respect for healthcare professionals and empathy for

---

1   Zhang Gaoxia, "From 'Appraisal Conclusions' to 'Appraisal Opinions,'" *Decision and Information Magazine*; "Proceedings of 'Decision Forum: Academic Symposium on the Application and Analysis of Management Decision Models,'" *Decision and Information Magazine* (2016):120–122.

2   Zhao Xiju, "Opinions of Medical Experts and Judges' Discretion in Medical Lawsuits: Who Is in Charge of Ups and Downs?," *Journal of Law and Medicine* 14, no. 3 (2007): 169–181.

patients. Although the statutory duty of care should always be the same, a clear shift has begun in recent years. Courts are increasingly hoping to force the medical industry to continuously improve itself and improve its work by raising the standard of duty of care. This is also in line with the development trend of modern civil law, which has moved from focusing on "case justice" to "social justice."

2. The court shall apply the judgment or mediation differently according to the specific case

In medical lawsuits, medical institutions and medical personnel often place great importance on the outcome of winning or losing a lawsuit because, in the public and medical industry conceptions, winning a case means not at fault, and losing a lawsuit means making a mistake. It seems that a civil judgment is a kind of moral judgment that is not black or white. As mentioned above, the standards for determining fault in civil torts are often forward-looking or forward-looking to a certain extent and do not necessarily negate the moral aspect of the tortfeasor. That is, it does not mean that a liable defendant should not be subjectively or morally condemned, but only that there is no necessarily corresponding relationship between subjective fault or morally reprehensible nature and negligence.[1] This requires the court to properly apply a "judgment" or "mediation" to close the case in future medical lawsuits. If medical personnel violate the current "medical and health management laws, administrative regulations, departmental rules, and diagnosis, treatment and nursing codes and practices" medical negligence, they should not settle the case through "mediation" but should pass a judgment to show the court's negative attitude towards medical negligence. However, if medical personnel have not violated "medical health management laws, administrative regulations, departmental regulations, and medical treatment and nursing standards and practices," but they have indeed not fulfilled the professionals' obligation to be careful, they should pass as much as possible. Settlement of the case through mediation.

---

1   Hu Xuemei, *British Tort Law* (Beijing: China University of Political Science and Law Press, 2008), 119.

3. The law accelerates the shift from "patriarchy" to "patient-centrism"

The current clinical situation in China is very similar to that in the UK 30 years ago. The idea that patients have the right to make their own decisions is often submerged in the rampant paternalism of the medical industry. Today, the mainstream slogan in the UK is no longer "Physicians Know You Best." "Doctor-patient partnership" is the slogan preferred by the current British government. In order to ensure the best interests of patients, the generally accepted principle is that physicians should negotiate rather than be arbitrary. This shift in ethical views is most clearly reflected in current industry and legal regulations, which require informed consent from patients who have the power to decide. Industry-specific regulations As the General Medical Council claims: "A successful doctor-patient relationship is built on trust. To build trust, patients' autonomy must be respected—it is up to them to decide whether to carry out a medical intervention. They must be provided with sufficient information in a way they can understand to enable them to make informed medical decisions."[1]

Just as the doctor will not simply think that what the physician has done is correct because of the view of "acting responsibly" and then win the case, the patient will also not simply win the case simply because of the view of "acting responsibly." In both cases, although the viewpoint of "responsible peers" is important, this viewpoint is not automatically equivalent to a legal conclusion. The judge has the power to identify and review the testimony of "responsible peers." Obviously, the shift from "patriarchy" to "patient-centrism," from medical experts monopolizing factual determination to judges intervening in factual determination, all made the medical industry feel very dissatisfied and difficult. Because litigation undoubtedly has a strong deterrent effect, making those working in clinical settings always vigilant.

The healthcare industry has always been like an independent kingdom, setting its own game rules. Judges are also very respectful of physicians. Physicians and other medical personnel are professionals who respect art

---

1   General Medical Council, "Seeking Patients' Consent: The Ethical Considerations," London: General Medical Council, 1999.

and science and possess important skills. The public trusts these disciplines, which are also very important to patients, and also means that healthcare workers are not the target of expensive and potentially damaging lawsuits. Therefore, judges have also allowed physicians to set their own industry standards and conduct collective professional evaluations to a large extent, as long as they are widely accepted by peers. This approach may not keep the standards very high; it may only be the minimum level that can be tolerated. However, this concept means that it is difficult for patients to prove that physicians' negligence is responsible; what is even more frightening is that the medical industry lacks the motivation to continuously improve and improve itself. Facts have shown that this attitude of high autonomy in the medical industry does not always set very high industry standards; on the contrary, it may simply be basic and not in line with the intent of national health policies, that is, standards that are in the best interest of patients. The traditional Chinese judicial position is also similar to the transformation that Britain is undergoing, from a position dominated by traditional medicine to a position dominated by the administration of justice. Although judges are still reluctant to challenge clinical standards easily, they seem more willing to challenge the physicians in individual cases, hoping that the industry's perspective will move closer to the position of judicial review.

Of course, there are negative effects. A creative physician has novel treatment methods and is unconventional. Although his expert peers support his approach, the physician may also be responsible for medical negligence if the judge sees arrogance, abnormal tests, or putting patients at unnecessary risk.

Legislative Improvement of Grounds of Justification in Medical Treatment in China Based on Xiao Zhijun's Case*

I. Informed Consent Not the Sole Grounds of Justification for Medical Actions

Grounds of justification, a key concept in civil law systems, refers to the fact that something that normally meets the elements of illegality is deemed not to be illegal due to the existence of other grounds. Generally speaking, grounds of justification include the following: justifiable defense, the act of rescue, negotiorum gestio, self-help, the justifiable performance of public duties, and consent of the victim. The grounds of justification for medical actions are mainly the following.

1. Consent of the victim (informed consent)

Medical treatment is often physically traumatic (i.e., unlawful), especially surgery, special examinations, or special treatments. For this reason, the law requires informed consent before the execution of a medical treatment

---

*   *Medicine and Philosophy (Humanistic & Social Medicine Edition)* 29, no. 2 (February 2008).

so that the traumatic effects of the treatment can be "prevented from being illegal."

Grounds of justification based on the patient's consent are premised on the fact that the medical institution and its medical staff must fulfill the duty of care to the patient in their medical activities. The duty of care is mainly the duty to explain, inform, and answer inquiries. If the medical institution and its medical personnel fail to fulfill the duty to explain, inform, answer inquiries or fulfill the duty to explain, inform, and answer imperfectly, they should be deemed to have failed to fulfill the duty of care reasonably, which may constitute a negligent tort. In this case, grounds of justification do not arise.

2. Act of rescue

Doctors generally categorize operations as emergency, non-emergency, or selective operations, depending on the needs and conditions of the patient. It is important to note that in this case, the doctor does not discuss with the patient's family the choice of a selective operation, but rather whether or not to resort to emergency operation upon being aware that the life of the pregnant woman and the fetus will be in jeopardy if the operation is not performed. Article 24 of the Law on Practicing Doctors of the People's Republic of China stipulates, "For patients in critical condition, physicians shall take urgent measures to treat them; they may not refuse emergency treatment." It is clear that the right of doctors to intervene in emergencies should be further clarified in future amendments to the law. If the patient is in an emergency, should there be de facto or express informed consent in order to prevent the violation of the law? In the author's opinion, it is obviously not.

Indeed, scholars have analyzed the grounds for justification of medical treatment at this point using different legal theories. Some scholars have suggested that it can be explained by the theory of implied consent. Implied consent means that, even in the absence of de facto or express consent, the plaintiff may be presumed to consent to certain (otherwise tortious) acts in certain special circumstances (e.g., emergency rescue). In these cases, the law assumes that the consent of the person concerned is implied because the benefit of the acts to the person concerned (e.g., the saving of life or the preservation of limbs) outweighs the loss to that person (e.g., the integrity of the body).[1] In this case, consent is indeed absent. Neither de facto nor express consent is available, and implied consent is only a legal assumption.

Other scholars believe that it should be explained by the justifiable performance of public duties.[2] However, the author does not agree with the idea of explaining the legitimacy of medical treatment with justifiable performance of public duties, since the justifiable performance of doctors' public duties should be strictly limited to the commissioning of legislation of public power.

In the case of emergency operations mentioned above, the legality of medical treatment should be interpreted in terms of the act of rescue. Such grounds of justification are established in Article 129 of the General Principles of the Civil Law of the People's Republic of China.

In this case, if the medical institution puts the life of the pregnant woman and her child in the first place and resuscitates her, there is no cause for criticism under the current laws of China. Furthermore, there is no need to worry about any lawsuits after the resuscitation because the Law on Practicing Doctors of the People's Republic of China and the Regulations on the Administration of Medical Institutions stipulate the obligation of medical institutions to rescue critically ill patients. Moreover, Article 129 of the General Principles of the Civil Law is a perfectly acceptable ground for an ex post facto defense.

3. Negotiorum gestio

There is also a legal relationship in medicine arising from de facto legal acts of a medical institution or a medical staff member towards a patient. According to the General Principles of the Civil Law, the negotiorum gestio of medical affairs refers to the behavior of a medical institution or a medical worker who voluntarily provides medical services to a patient in order to prevent the patient's life and health interests from being jeopardized in the absence of a contractual obligation or a legal obligation.

---

1   Vincent R. Johnson, *Mastering Torts: A Student's Guide to the Law of Torts* (Beijing: China Renmin University Press, 2004), 44–45.

2   Yang Lixin, *Tort Law* (Shanghai: Fudan University Press, 2005), 122–123.

Is it a violation of the Law on Practicing Doctors of the People's Republic of China for medical personnel who discover a patient outside a hospital and fail to treat him or her? Without the presence of a guardian, does the hospital have the obligation to treat a patient who is incapacitated and in a "non-urgent condition"? In the author's opinion, the above behavior should be interpreted with negotiorum gestio in accordance with the General Principles of the Civil Law. In this way, it can also alleviate the duty of care in the management process by the bona fide administrator and alleviate or exempt the damage caused by their management behavior to the person being managed.

4. Official conduct

Based on the special nature of medical treatment and the protection of people's lives and physical health, the state legally confers on medical institutions or medical personnel the obligation to provide compulsory treatment and on patients to receive compulsory treatment. It is a special case in the legal relationship in medicine, which constitutes the exercise of public power. In other words, the medical institution or medical personnel serve as the user or agent of the state, and the legal relationship in medicine stands between the state and the patient, which can be called the compulsory medical relationship. In this case, the doctor's official conduct becomes a ground of justification.[1] For example, such provisions are set forth in the Law on Prevention and Control of Infectious Diseases and the Law of the People's Republic of China on Mental Health.

II. The Key to This Case Being Whether the Intent to Refuse Surgery Is Genuine and Valid

Informed consent is legally valid only if the patient's declaration of intention to consent (or not to consent) is genuine. In fact, the future focus of the dispute between the plaintiff and the defendant will be on this issue.

---

1   Wang Liming, *Research on Tort Law* (Beijing: China Renmin University Press, 2004), 554–555.

The declaration of intention means that the actor makes its intention of the inner effect of a civil legal act expressed externally in a certain way and known to others and exerts some binding effect.[1] For civil law countries, an error in declaration of intent has traditionally been based on an internal logical structure that strictly distinguishes between errors of expression and errors of motive. This case should be about the latter—error of motive.

As far as civil law countries are concerned, in the traditional sense, they make a strict distinction between the error of motive and the error of declaration and regard it as one of the usual patterns of the error of declaration of intention.[2] According to Wang Zejian, an error of motive is an error in the cause of a declaration of intention. It refers to the incorrect recognition of the fact that the intention of the representor is significant in the process of formation of his/her intention for determining a particular content of the intention. Since the motives are hidden in the heart of the individual and cannot be seen by others, the representor is unlikely to be allowed to revoke it at will in order to prevent jeopardizing the safety of public transactions. In other words, the risk of a mistake in the formation of the intention is borne by the representor. So, does it affect the validity of the declaration of intention if the counterparty is aware of the mistake in the motive of the representor? In principle, the answer is negative based on the general knowledge. The reason is that the counterparty is aware of the cause and the error of the representor's intention based on the declaration, but it is still insufficient to transfer the risk of the representor's mistake of anticipation or failure of speculation. It is only when the counterparty has contracted by taking advantage of the erroneous motive of the representor in violation of the principle of good faith that the counterparty is deemed to have abused its rights and is not protected.[3] An error of motive is an incorrect conception

---

1   Zhang Junhao, *Principles of Civil Law* (Beijing: China University of Political Science and Law Press, 1997), 209.

2   Wang Zejian, *The General Principles of Civil Law* (Beijing: China University of Political Science and Law Press, 2001), 371–373.

3   Ibid., 376.

or understanding by the representor of certain situations that are of great significance to his decision to express this intention.[1]

In the field of medicine, if the medical practitioner fails to inform the patient of his/her condition, the available treatments, or the advantages and disadvantages of the various treatments in sufficient detail and in layman's terms, the patient's consent or disagreement should be invalidated in accordance with the law. However, in this case, we must strictly examine whether or not the medical practitioner knows that an error of motive has been made in the representor's declaration of intention. If the medical practitioner cannot judge that the patient's expression of intention is wrong, he should be exempted from civil liability; on the contrary, he should be investigated for civil liability. In the case of Xiao Zhijun, Xiao Zhijun expressed his intention of "refusing cesarean section operation at his own risk" (whether he also expressed his intention of saving the lives of his wife and child, and whether he refused to sign for fear that the hospital would exempt itself from liability and he would assume excessive responsibility, should be the key facts to be examined by the judge). If the judge concludes that the medical practitioner is unable to determine that the patient's expression of intent is incorrect after reviewing the facts, the medical practitioner should be exempted from civil liability. On the contrary, the medical practitioner should be held civilly liable.

III. Amendment Needed to Article 33 of the Regulations on the Administration of Medical Institutions

The author believes that the revision of the Regulations on the Administration of Medical Institutions is imperative, and it is urgent to change the "ambiguous" conditions and clarify the therapeutic privilege.

---

1   Karl Larenz, *The General Theory of the German Civil Law*, trans. Wang Xiaoye and Shao Jiandong, vol. 1 (Beijing: Law Press China, 2003), 504, 524.

Normally, the general rights of the physician are subordinated to the rights of the patient, which is the fundamental requirement for the realization of the patient's freedom and autonomy. However, in extremely specific cases, it is necessary to limit the patient's right to autonomy and to fulfill the physician's own will, so that the physician can fulfill his obligations to the patient and be responsible for the patient's fundamental rights and interests. This right is called therapeutic privilege. In the 1993 case of Korman V. Mallina, Judge Moore of the Supreme Court of the State of Alaska, in his judgment, defined the circumstances of therapeutic privilege: (1) when full and complete disclosure of viable alternative treatments and their consequences would adversely affect the patient's physical or mental health; (2) when the patient lacks the capacity to express consent due to insanity or minority; and (3) when the physician's duty to inform is thwarted by the emergence of a critical or emergency situation, and it is impractical to obtain the patient's consent (Korman V. Mallina, 25 P2d 1145, Supreme). In the author's opinion, the legislation in China should be explicitly supplemented with the following circumstances of therapeutic privilege.

1. Refusal of treatment by the patient

In general, the patient has the right to refuse treatment, but such refusal can only be exercised if the patient has made a rational decision, the law permits it, and the physician has made clear the advantages and disadvantages of such refusal, and if such refusal is in line with public order and good custom. However, the attending physician should exercise the right of special intervention on the following special occasions: (1) when the refusal of treatment might lead to serious consequences or irremediable damage to the patient; (2) when such a decision is made by a person who is incapable of conduct or has limited capacity to act; (3) when such a decision is made by a patient who is in a state of extreme emotional instability; (4) when such a decision is made by drugs that have an effect on the thinking and cognitive capacities of the patient; and (5) in cases specifically prescribed by the legislation.

2. Experimental treatment of humans

Some highly dangerous experiments, or experiments that may cause death or disability, might be intervened in due course, even if the patient agrees to them for certain purposes, such as the desire to be cured of a disease, especially a disease for which no effective treatment is available, through experiments that may be effective, even though they are risky; or if the patient agrees to them for purely financial considerations but the doctor concludes that the patient is not in a fit state to undergo the highly dangerous medical experiments through examinations. The medical experiment shall be discontinued or suspended if necessary to protect the patient's interests.

3. Necessary behavioral control

Doctors can exercise their right to intervene in patients with psychiatric disorders in the course of a seizure and in patients with certain diseases prescribed by law, such as AIDS, leprosy, and other virulent infectious diseases. Doctors may force patients to be hospitalized and receive medical treatment by taking reasonable, effective, temporary, and moderate coercive measures in accordance with the law.

4. Resuscitation of suicidal patients

A patient who commits suicide is brought to a hospital for emergency treatment. If the patient apparently refuses medical treatment based on the suicide, the doctor must provide adequate and timely resuscitation to such a critical patient.

This case teaches us a profound lesson: we can no longer formulate our laws with a "patriarchal" mindset. We can no longer take the choice of the "head of the household" for granted as the choice of every member of that household. And beyond that, we can no longer set our laws in a "culture of ambiguity."

Control of Fetal Sex Identification for Non-medical Needs: A Case Study of Fetal Portraits

I. Controversy over "Fetal Portrait"[1]

Almost all parents shoot a photo album for their newborn babies in a photo studio to record their children's beautiful and innocent childhood memories. But recently, it has become popular in many cities in China to take a "fetal portrait" of the baby still in the womb using three-dimensional ultrasound technology, and it has become fashionable among "mothers-to-be." As a result, memories of the pre-birth period have been added to many children's photo albums. For 200 *yuan*, a hospital can take photos and videos of a baby who has yet to be born. At a maternal and child care service center in Shanghai, physicians can take a picture of the baby in the womb while examining the pregnant woman, using a dynamic three-dimensional ultrasound diagnostic system. Expectant parents can then take home portraits of their babies still in the womb. The reporter learned from a dozen expectant mothers who had their "portraits" taken that most of them knew the sex of their children. "We can approach our acquaintances and put in a good word,

1. Supported by the Program of the National Population and Family Planning Commission on "Research on Legal Issues Related to Fetal Sex Identification and Pregnancy Termination"; *Chinese Hospital Management*, no. 26 (April 2006).

and they will generally tell us the sex of the baby." "The ultrasound images are very precise, and we can almost tell the sex of the baby ourselves."

According to the hospitals, in principle, photographs are only taken of fetuses above six months of age, and only the head of the fetus is photographed, not the lower part of the fetus where the sex can be identified. When pregnant women undergo color Doppler ultrasound examinations, physicians are not allowed to tell the parents about the sex of the fetus, even though they know that. If individual parents-to-be ask for sex identification in violation of the regulations, doctors will not hesitate to refuse. On the other hand, some other scholars suggest that fetal portrait is trying to exploit the loopholes of the legal system of gender identification in China and should be prohibited, investigated, and dealt with.

II. Legal System of Fetal Sex Identification in China

1. Current legal provisions on fetal sex identification

China's legislation on fetal sex identification is firstly in the Law of the People's Republic of China on Maternal and Infant Health Care. Article 23 of the Measures for Implementation of the Law of the People's Republic of China on Maternal and Infant Health Care further clarifies the relevant provisions. It stipulates that "Where a fetus is suspected of contracting sex-linked genetic diseases, therefore gender identification is needed, such gender identification shall be made by a medical and healthcare institution designated by the administrative department of public health of the people's government of the province, autonomous region or municipality directly under the Central Government in accordance with the provisions of the administrative department of the health of the State Council."[1]

In 2002, the National Family Planning Commission, the Ministry of Health, and the National Medical Products Administration promulgated the

---

1   Li Luyun, "Fetal Sex Identification and Its Significance," *Chinese Journal of Practical Gynecology and Obstetrics* 15, no. 7 (1999): 398–400.

Provisions on Prohibiting Fetal Sex Identification for Non-medical Needs and Sex-Selective Pregnancy Termination. Article 6 clearly stipulates that the implementation of fetal sex identification for medical needs shall be reviewed collectively by a panel of experts consisting of more than three persons from the implementing organization. If, upon diagnosis, the pregnancy must be terminated, the implementing organization shall issue a medical diagnosis report and notify the administrative department of family planning of the people's government at the county level of the medical diagnosis results.

In China, all forms of sex determination for all purposes are illegal, except for those specified in Article 23 of the Measures for Implementation of the Law of the People's Republic of China on Maternal and Infant Health Care.

2. Legal analysis of "fetal portraits"

In the author's opinion, the law prohibits fetal sex identification, while the hospital provides fetal portrait photography. There are some conceptual differences between the two. However, from the analysis of the results, it should be concluded that the hospital's practice of "fetal portrait," in which the whole body of the fetus is photographed, is apparently against the law.

The development of science and technology has made it possible for three-dimensional ultrasound to clearly show the image of the fetus. When the general public can make judgments about gender on the basis of such images, such technological development has actually replaced the subjective judgment of medical science, or even made it more accurate than the subjective judgment of medical science. Even if the doctor does not reveal his/her judgment when providing the medical image, the gender of the fetus can be identified as long as the fetal portrait reflects the sex of the fetus.

Under the rule of law, there are three modes of human behavior: the mode of what can be done, the mode of what should be done, and the mode of what should not be done. Everything which is not allowed is forbidden; everything which is not forbidden is allowed. However, when some people do something prohibited by the law for some illegal interests, they always juggle with words in the law first. In fact, it is not feasible to circumvent the law by using differences in words. Although legal provisions cannot be all-encompassing, the law's application principle is that what is clearly stipulated must be strictly observed, and what is not clearly stipulated must comply with legal principles and the spirit or purpose of the legislation. For this reason, although there may be loopholes in the law, it is still possible to judge the legal nature of such acts by applying the principles of the law and in accordance with the original intent of the legislation. Legality requires not only that the means be lawful, but also that the purpose in question be lawful. A civil act that uses legal means to cover up an illegal purpose is an invalid civil act, which also has illegal consequences with the parties concerned being punished by the law.

Even as the medical institution states, "in principle, only the head of the fetus is photographed, not the lower part where the sex can be identified." The author personally believes that such behavior is against the non-profit nature of public medical institutions and the national regulations on the price management of medical services, so it is not advisable to provide such services.

III. Reasons for Strictly Prohibiting Fetal Sex Identification for Non-medical Needs

Before the 1980s, the sex ratio at birth in China was basically within the normal range (its sex ratio at birth usually fluctuated between 102 and 107). However, since the 1980s, the sex ratio at birth in China has risen significantly. In 1982, the sex ratio at birth of the third population census was 108.1500, which was the first sign of a high ratio. It rose to 111.13 in the fourth census in 1990 and reached 116.9 in the fifth census in 2000. It has been significantly higher than the internationally recognized sex ratio at birth (103.100–106.100). A comparison of the results of the 2000 Population Census with the results of previous censuses and 1% sample surveys shows that the high sex ratio at birth in China has not abated, but has continued to rise in recent years.[1]

---

1 Wang Mengzhang, "Thoughts on the Governance of Sex Ratio at Birth," *Chinese Public Administration*, no. 2 (2005): 32–33.

If the current high sex ratio of the population at birth does not change, or even continues to increase, a very frightening situation will arise in the years to come. In other words, in each age group of young and middle-aged people, the male population outnumbers the female population by 12% to 15%. According to the Fifth Population Census, the male population in the age group of 0–4 years is 37.65 million, which is 20.2% more than the female population of 31.33 million. If calculated on the basis of the current sex ratio at birth and birth rate, there will be about 300 million males and 250 million females under the age of 40 by the year 2040, with 50 million more males than females. Given the influence of the Chinese view that men are older than women in choosing their spouses and the fact that some women are celibate and do not get married, there will be at least 30 million men in the age group of 21 to 40 years who may experience greater difficulties in their marriage.

This situation, in reality, has at least several harmful effects: (1) The male population in each age group of the population under 40 years of age out-numbers the female population by more than 1 million on average, which will inevitably lead to pressure on marriages. As a result, it may increase social instability. (2) Since females are the mainstay of population reproduc-tion, a decrease in the female population will hinder population reproduc-tion, lead to an imbalance in the population's age structure, and aggravate the degree of population aging. (3) The surplus of the male population may further have a "squeezing effect" on the employment of females, and the reduction of employment opportunities for females may directly affect the promotion of their status. (4) The decrease in the female population will lead to the shrinkage of the child and adolescent population and the increase in the elderly population. As a result, the demand for consumption will be weakened, affecting economic growth in turn.

IV. Improvement of the Legal System of Fetal Sex Identification for Non-medical Needs in China

1. Solving the ideological problems from the root cause

One of the fundamental causes of the imbalance in the sex ratio at birth is the influence and constraints of traditional fertility concepts. It is still a long-term and arduous task to change the public's concept of reproduction. We should strengthen the construction of schools for the population, increase the scientific and technological content of publicity and education programs, and intensify publicity and education efforts, especially to explain and publicize the harmful effects of the imbalance in the sex ratio at birth on society. At the same time, the "New Style of Marriage and Childbearing in All Families" campaign should be carried out in depth to enable farmers to gradually establish a new concept of marriage and childbearing. In addition to regulating people's reproductive behaviors through the rules and regulations of government departments and the laws of the country, it is also necessary to create a publicity atmosphere by means of formats that are pleasing to the public, such as movies, television, radio, and other cultural and artistic programs, so as to advocate a correct reproductive culture and promote a change in attitudes.

2. Improving the social security system and using benefits as a guide to encourage the female population of childbearing age to give up their preference for having boys

After nearly 30 years of efforts, China's family planning policy has become deeply rooted in people's minds. However, due to the constraints of the level of development of productive forces, there is still a big gap between some people's desire to have children and the national birth policy. Therefore, in reality, the state should set up a necessary social security system for families practicing family planning and apply relevant preferential policies, so that families practicing family planning can truly feel politically honored and financially benefited. In addition, the state should help solve the difficulties in production and life of some rural families with family planning due to the shortage of male labor force and offer necessary support to them, so as to demonstrate the fairness and justice of society.[1]

3. Perfecting the current laws

At present, there is no other effective provision to address the liability of those who illegally introduce and organize pregnant women to undergo fetal sex determination for non-medical needs or sex-selective pregnancy termination operations. Provisions in this regard should also be refined. For those who do not have the qualification to practice medicine but engage in illegal identification of fetal sex and illegal pregnancy termination, some scholars suggest that the criminal liabilities for such acts can be pursued with the crimes of illegal practice of medicine and sabotage of family planning as specified in the Criminal Law. As for the criminal responsibility of persons who are qualified for prenatal diagnosis but engage in illegal fetal sex identification and illegal termination of pregnancy,[2] the author personally does not favor amending the Criminal Law of the People's Republic of China to add more crimes for such illegal acts. Instead, consideration should be given to imposing greater administrative liability on offenders, especially through the mechanism of "lifetime prohibition of employment," in order to heighten the cost of violating the law.

4. Establishing a system of administrative incentives

Due to the mobility of people and the means of surveillance in modern society, administrative organs do not have sufficient human and material resources to collect clues in cases. They are thus unable to investigate and deal with the cases efficiently. For the solution of this problem, it is doubtlessly the best footnote to describe it as "the masses have sharp eyes." Whatever the motivation for reporting, the conditions for rewarding reporting should

---

1   Tang Jun, "The Essence of Sex Ratio Imbalance in Inadequate Social Security," *Social Observation*, no. 3 (2005): 23.

2   Xu Wenping, "Certain Issues in Combating the Imbalance in the Sex Ratio at Birth and Amending the Criminal Law," *Population and Family Planning*, no. 6 (2005): 24–27.

be made known to the public, and the rewards should be strictly honored. Confidentiality should be kept for whistleblowers. At the same time, reporting channels should be improved, and telephone and Internet reporting channels similar to 12315 should be set up. In addition, all reports should be responded to, emphasizing the report's effectiveness. Citizens should be motivated to report illegal fetal sex identification, sex-selective pregnancy termination surgery, and the illegal sale or use of drugs for pregnancy termination. As seen in other aspects of administrative law enforcement where administrative reward systems have been established, this system has been designed to work very well, and it allows for the establishment of an efficient channel on top of the active supervision by the supervisory authorities.

5. Enhancing information sharing among regulatory authorities

Due to the multiplicity of regulatory departments, despite the mutual information dissemination system, it is observed that each department is responsible for its respective tasks due to the lack of smooth channels. In view of this, it is necessary to establish a linkage system. For example, if the drug supervision department detects cases of illegal sale of drugs for termination of pregnancy, it should inform the health department and the family planning department in a timely manner, so that the other departments can investigate and deal with the case in a prompt and timely manner based on the clues.

6. Blocking the illegal exit of illegal sex identification

Blocking the illegal exit of illegal sex identification is an important measure to address such social problems. The main reason for the social dangerousness of illegal sex identification is the selective pregnancy termination after identification. For this reason, legislation should be adopted to strictly limit the practice of termination of pregnancy by artificial means. Some people may worry that such a provision is contrary to China's family planning policy. According to the 2001 Law of the People's Republic of China on Population and Family Planning, the legal consequences of violating the state's family planning policy are only the payment of social maintenance fees and partial administrative responsibility stipulated in Article 41. That is to say, we can impose strict limits at the point of pregnancy termination, and then gender identification would not be socially harmful. In fact, Article 7 of Provisions on Prohibiting Fetal Sex Identification for Non-medical Needs and Sex-Selective Pregnancy Termination has already made restrictions on such cases. In other words, if a person meets the fertility conditions stipulated in the regulations on population and family planning of provinces, autonomous regions, and municipalities directly under the central government, has received a birth service certificate, and intends to undergo surgery for termination of pregnancy in the middle term or above (more than 14 weeks of gestation) for non-medical needs, she must be approved by the administrative department for family planning of the People's Government at the county level, or by the family planning agency of the local township (town) people's government, or of the local subdistrict office, and must be granted the corresponding certificate. However, the provisions of Article 7 are not explicit enough, and the degree of control to be exercised by the administrative department of family planning remains unclear. It is suggested that legislation should be enacted to specify the conditions for restricting the termination of pregnancy for those pregnant women who have exceeded the 14th week of gestation. It can be stipulated that pregnancy termination is prohibited unless it is justified by one of the following circumstances: (1) One of the circumstances prohibiting marriage stipulated in Article 7 of the Marriage Law of the People's Republic of China occurs. (2) The pregnant woman or her spouse is suffering from a hereditary, contagious, or mental disease that hinders eugenics. (3) The continuation of gestation constitutes a great danger to the woman's body or health. (4) The fetus is malformed or suffers from a serious hereditary disease. (5) The fetus is mentally retarded or suffers from other severe defects. (6) The termination of pregnancy is requested by the victim of coercive sexual intercourse. (7) The termination of pregnancy is requested by a young girl under 16 years of age. (8) The termination is requested by a person whose psychological health or family life will be affected by the pregnancy or childbirth. (9) The termination of pregnancy is requested in violation of the laws and regulations of the state on population and family planning.

Philosophy Reflection from Modern Psychiatry to Post-Psychiatry

Today, many countries, led by the United Kingdom, have begun to alter the nature of the mental health industry by adapting their national policies and legislation. For solutions to the links between poverty, unemployment, and mental disorders, national policies and legislation have begun to focus on vulnerable groups and social exclusion.[1] The importance of social environments, value systems, and collaborative working has been emphasized in the policy and legal frameworks of national mental health services in various countries. This change is undoubtedly a rethinking and a challenge to modern psychiatry under the traditional biomedical model.[2] In short, there is a desire from the government and the public to revolutionize the relationship between psychiatry and its practitioners and clients. As Muir Gray argues, this need is not only specific to modern psychiatry, but to all medical specialties. The public's faith in science and technology, which was one of the most important features of the 20th century, is gradually fading.[3]

According to Muir Gray, the mission of the postmodern medical industry is not only to maintain and enhance its achievements in the modern era, but also to adjust to the development of the postmodern society. Its focus

---

1 Department of Health, *Saving Lives: Our Healthier Nation* (London: Stationery Office, 1998).

2 Department of Health, *Modern Standards and Service Models: Mental Health* (London: Stationery Office, 1999).

3 Muir Gray J. A., "Postmodern Medicine," *Lancet*, no. 354 (1999): 1550–1553.

should shift from "phenomenal evidence" to "value systems," and its area of interest from "profit" to "challenging itself." The medical profession has recognized this change and begun to accept it. However, in the domain of mental health, there is another difficulty that other medical specialties will never face, and the achievements made by it in the 20th century are also doubted. For example, while people have complained about long waiting times in hospitals, bad attitudes of healthcare providers, and ineffective communication between doctors and patients, few people have questioned the technology of medicine itself. Psychiatry in the 20th century had been challenged and questioned by the public.[1] It is impossible to imagine that the public would launch an "anti-pediatric" or "critical psychiatry" movement. However, the movements of "anti-psychiatry" and "critical psychiatry" have a long history. Psychiatry in the 20th century has resisted these challenges conservatively and has established its medical identity. Although the discipline survived the opposition movement of the 1860s, fundamental problems in its ethical and legal aspects remain unresolved.

I. Origins and Reflections of Modern Psychiatry

From the very beginning, at both ends of psychiatry, it is not the doctor and the patient but the whole society and the excluded party. Society was in the hands of the majority, represented by the powerful; the patients with mental illness were a minority, not capable of resisting the oppression of society. At that time, the power to speak and act in society was in the hands of a very small number of influential figures. Although the psychiatric activities of patients with mental illness could be understood by the outside world, they were ruthlessly discarded and suppressed by the majority because of the apparent conflict of interest with the dominant group. It was a direct oppression of the individual's body by power.

The modern psychiatry of mankind has its roots in the European Enlightenment, stemming from people's pursuit and exploration of reason and individual will in the Enlightenment. The postmodernist reflection on it is

---

1   T. Szasz, *The Myth of Mental Illness* (New York: Harper and Row, 1961).

not to resist the influence and role of the Enlightenment, but rather to re-mind people not to overlook its dangers while recognizing its merits and to be cautious about its "progressiveness." We must recognize that science and technology may liberate people, but they can also be tools to deprive dissent-ers of their right to speak. On the one hand, the European Enlightenment's quest for reason and order led to a society where every effort was made to exclude the "irrational" heretics. As Roy Porter puts it in his book *A Social History of Madness: Stories of the Insane*, from the 17th century onwards, out of a zeal for reason, it became the task of society to criticize, condemn, and even repress those who were deemed stupid or irrational by the ruling class or the dominant group of people in the society. These individuals were judged to be detrimental to the development of society and even a threat.[1] Foucault, in particular, argued that the proliferation of mental asylums was not a result of advances in medicine, but rather a form of social ostracism. Psychiatry arose directly from these behaviors.[2] Roy Porter holds a similar view, "The establishment of asylums gave birth to psychiatry. It was only when and if large numbers of patients with mental illnesses were institution-alized in the asylums that psychiatry had a real chance to develop. On the other hand, the belief in reason led people to be convinced that the best way to deal with mental disorders was only through medicine."[3] Starting with Descartes, the Enlightenment was also concerned with the development of individual consciousness. As a result, phenomenology and psychoanalysis emerged. However, in the 20th century, psychiatry did not critically accept the emphasis on reason and the individual's will.

1. Mental disorder as an internal problem

One of the most influential psychiatric works of the 20th century was Karl Jasper's *General Psychopathology*. Jasper made the external manifestations of

1   R. Porter, *A Social History of Madness: Stories of the Insane* (London: Weidenfeld and Nicolson, 1987).

2   M. Foucault, ed., *Madness and Civilization: A History of Insanity in the Age of Reason*, trans. Liu B. C. and Yang Y. Y. (SDX Joint Publishing Company, 2004), 63–66.

3   R. Porter, *A Social History of Madness: Stories of the Insane* (London: Weidenfeld and Nicolson, 1987).

mental disorder independent of its intrinsic nature: "Although the psychology of the person concerned is of some importance in describing the events of mental disorder, we are only interested in their external manifestations from a phenomenological point of view."[1] These views profoundly influenced the development of psychiatry in Europe and around the world. Since then, psychiatry has remained oblivious to the contextual background of psychological phenomena. Mental disorders and depression have been defined as abnormal personal experiences and feelings. Social and environmental factors are considered to be of little or no significance. It is partly because that the majority of mental health cases occur in hospitals, and that regimens are based on pharmacological or psychotherapeutic treatment of the individual patient. It is also partly because the analysis of the cases focuses on the patient at the physiological, behavioral, cognitive, and psychodynamic levels.

2. Scientific explanations of mental disorder

The Enlightenment claimed that human suffering could be eliminated through the advancement of reason and science, and the function of psychiatry was to establish an understanding of mental disorders within the framework of pathology and neuroscience while excluding the spiritual, ethical, and political factors. This phenomenon has recently culminated in the Decade of the Brain program, which claims that mental disorders are caused by dysfunctions of the nervous system and that they can be cured by medication at specific neurological sites. Nowadays, those who question this doctrine can almost be regarded as heretics and even labeled as anti-scientific.

The Diagnostic and Statistical Manual of Mental Disorders (DSM) of the United States of America also describes psychological problems in scientific and technical terms. More than 300 types of mental disorders are defined in the manual, most of which have been defined and included in the last 20 years. Kuichins and Kirk, who were responsible for the program, stated that "the DSM has guided us to take a new look at psychiatric manifestations such as depression, anxiety, sexual behavior, alcohol and drug dependence,

---

1   K. Jasper, *General Psychopathology* (Manchester: Manchester University Press, 1963).

and many other behaviors. Ultimately, the DSM changed our perceptions of important social events and organizations."[1] The history of insanity has made us concerned about the current state and trends of the DSM ...

In 1851, American physician Samuel Cartwright published an article in the *New Orleans Medical and Surgical Journal* about "drapetomania," a disease that was then directed at black slaves and which manifested itself in the tendency of black slaves to run away from the estates of their white masters. Homosexuality was included as a mental disorder in the first edition of the DSM in 1952. It was further recognized as a mental illness in the second edition of the DSM in 1968. In 1973, there was a debate within the American Psychiatric Association about whether homosexuality was a mental disorder. In the end, those in favor of removing homosexuality from mental disorders won by a narrow margin. Today, most European countries still recognize fetishism as a mental disorder and describe it as sexual arousal and gratification by relying on certain inanimate objects. Many fetishes are extensions of the human body, such as lingerie and high heels. A person can be diagnosed as a fetishist if he or she experiences periodic, intense sexual desires and fantasies about these objects for more than six months, and if they are a significant source of sexual stimulus. Will fetishism still be a mental disorder in 15 or 30 years?[2]

3. Psychiatry and oppressiveness

Although psychiatry became therapeutic during the Enlightenment era, it was still associated with social ostracism, incarceration, and so on. However, this seems to have been an improvement on the punitive internment that preceded it. The mentally ill were labeled as "insane" and forced to mentally accept this status. The real insanity was not the abnormal behavior at the beginning, but the confusion and fear of being given an identity. In the 20th century, when psychiatry claimed to have a medical solution to mental dis-

---

1   Kutchins H. and Kirk S., *Making Us Crazy: DSM: The Psychiatric Bible and the Creation of Mental Disorders* (London: Constable, 1999).

2   T. Hope., ed., *Medical Ethics: A Very Short Introduction*, trans. Wu J. H. and Li F. (Yilin Press, 2010), 73–74.

orders, the public began to accept the role of science and technology. Legislation gave the medical profession a great deal of power, and psychiatrists had the power and duty to detain patients forcibly, administering powerful medications and electro-convulsive therapies. Medicine seems to have provided the legislative basis and evidence for these coercive medical legislations. Today, the socially oppressive nature of the profession has only recently been addressed within the psychiatry community. Most psychiatrists have made great efforts to eliminate the distinction between themselves and practitioners of other medical professions. It has recently been reported that psychiatrists want to equate mental disorders with other physical illnesses in legislation.

With the evolution of modernity, the way in which reason is arbitrary has also changed. In today's society, reason is more represented as a conspirator than as a despot.[1] Instead of arbitrarily rejecting or suppressing irrationality as dissent, it keeps them under firm control by various gentle methods, mainly normative models, so as to bring them consciously back to the order of reason. Under the influence of the Enlightenment, the oppression of the mentally ill in society was transformed from outright rejection in the Middle Ages to hypocritical hypocrisy. Patients with mental illness went from physical torture to mental suffering, which was more ethereal and more deeply embedded in the inner nuances of the mind. It may not seem so surprising, and it is within most people's ethical boundaries, so this therapeutic privilege model has been functioning well. However, the oppression of power behind this phenomenon is much more than that. The oppression of minorities by majorities and of disadvantaged groups by dominant groups pervades every corner of life, and it wears a thicker and more ornate mask.

---

1   Yang D. C., "Modernity and the Fate of the Other: Foucault's Critical Analysis of the Relationship between Reason and Non-reason," *Social Sciences in Nanjing*, no. 6 (2001): 1–7.

II. Vision and Principles of Post-Psychiatry

1. The importance of context

The social, political, and cultural contexts should be the key to identifying mental disorders.[1] I believe that mental health interventions need not be centered on the individual patient's medical diagnosis and treatment. It does not mean denying the importance of the biological perspective, but rather shifting the primary focus to the contextual environment in which the biological characteristics arise. Events, responses, and social networks can never be analyzed or measured separately. They are interconnected through meaningful connections that can be explored and elucidated, even if these connections cannot be explained in simple terms.

2. Changing psychiatry from a science-oriented to a humanistic approach

Clinical effectiveness and outcome-oriented therapies are the mainstay of medicine today, suggesting that clinical practice should be dominated by science. Psychiatry has also tried to address its dilemmas in this way. However, the problem is that it overlooks the importance of personal value systems in both research and clinical practice. All medical practice is concerned with certain assumptions and values, and psychiatry is concerned with assumptions and values in the clinical setting because it is primarily an investigation of beliefs, emotions, interpersonal relationships, and behaviors. Some medical anthropologists and philosophers have pointed out the assumptions and values that constitute the basis for the categorization of mental disorders.[2]

---

1   R. Rorty, *Philosophy and the Mirror of Nature* (Princeton: Princeton University Press, 1979).

2   A. Gaines, *Ethnopsychiatry: The Cultural Construction of Professional and Folk Psychiatries* (Albany: State University of New York Press, 1992).

3. Re-examining the social oppressiveness of mental disorders

Some truths seem self-evident to everyone. It is no doubt an advance of civilization that there have been moves from the banishment and expulsion of the insane to their institutionalization for care in asylums and to the creation of modern psychiatric institutions, which provide for a comfortable life and careful treatment of the insane. It is more than a sign of humanity to replace arbitrariness and brutality with evidence-based justice and mercy, from public torture to solitary confinement. This is how we have always looked at society and judged history. Yet, Foucault remarks that these things, which have always been taken for granted and are innate to us, have all been shaped and produced by power. They are like a vicious joke, like an absurd truth. His writings on the history of madness and prisons reveal to us how that mysterious power has devoured mankind. The so-called advancement of history is nothing but a self-adjustment of the workings of power. He tells us that insanity is not a natural phenomenon, but a product of civilization. "There can be no history of insanity if there is no history of cultures that have characterized this phenomenon as madness and persecuted it." The diminution of the severity of punishment is nothing but a shift of the object of punishment from the body to the spirit, as it no longer causes physical suffering but deprives the freedom of the spirit. It is thus "the history of the interrelationship between the modern soul and a new power of judgment." In both cases, it embodies a transmutation of power: the elevation of power from the subjugation of the body to the control of the mind.

The debate about the new mental health movement in Britain has led us to re-examine the relationship between medicine and mental disorders. Many of the clients have questioned the medical model and are therefore dissatisfied with the policy of forced institutionalization in this movement. It does not mean that society cannot deprive any person with a mental disorder of his or her liberty. However, out of a questioning of the neutrality and objectivity of modern psychiatry, post-psychiatry rejects the dominant role of the medical approach in treatment.[1] Mechanisms to prevent social

---

1   N. Eastman, "Mental Health Law: Civil Liberties and the Principle of Reciprocity," *BMJ* 308 (1994): 43.

oppressiveness must be established in the legislation, with doctors being entitled to request the compulsory institutionalization of a patient, but not to make the final decision. Even in the initial decision-making process of institutionalization, non-medical professionals should be involved and preside over the decision-making process.

III. Conclusion

Post-psychiatry has attempted to break away from the conflict between the psychiatry community and the anti-psychiatry community. The anti-psychiatry community has criticized psychiatry for being oppressive and for being founded on a false medical ideology. It is committed to freeing the mentally ill from its clutches. Similarly, the psychiatry community criticizes the anti-psychiatry community for being guided by a false ideology. Both sides are convinced that mental disorders can and should be properly analyzed and understood.[1] Post-psychiatry opposes this view. Although it does not propose new ideas about mental disorders, it offers a variety of perspectives. Most importantly, it insists on a client-centered approach to psychiatry. Post-psychiatry differs from anti-psychiatry in its therapeutic approach. It does not seek to replace the vital role of medical technology with other therapies. It is not intended to present a set of firm ideas and concepts, but rather a guidepost to help us move forward.

Like other disciplines in medicine, psychiatry must adapt to what Muir Gray has called the "postmodern environment." Mental health practices are faced with difficulties within the framework of modernism. More and more psychiatrists have turned their attention to the philosophical (ethical), historical, anthropological, and legal aspects of the discipline. In fact, precisely because psychiatry has always been controversial, it can adapt to the postmodern society more than any other field of medicine. Postmodern psychiatrists seek to emancipate mental health services and promote their development by addressing contexts, value systems, and group solidarity.

---

1 P. Bracken, "Beyond Liberation: Michel Foucault and the Notion of a Critical Psychiatry," *Philos Psychiatry Psychol*, no. 2 (1995): 1–13.

Rethinking of the Dangerousness Principle of Compulsory Treatment to Mental Disorders

I. Definition of Dangerousness Principle

The dangerousness principle is integral to mental health law in many developed countries or regions. Stringent dangerousness principles are also provided for in the mental health laws of some states of the United States, Australia, and most European countries,[1] as well as in countries or regions such as Israel, Russia, Canada, and Taiwan, China.[2] For example, according to German law, compulsory medical treatment is only allowed for persons with mental disorders when their illness poses a significant risk of harm to themselves, others, or public safety and cannot be eliminated by other means.[3]

Prior to the 1960s, it was legally mandated that patients be committed to an asylum for a lunatic solely pursuant to a mental illness requiring treat-

1   H. Dressing and H. J. Salize, "Compulsory Admission of Mentally Ill Patients in European Union Member States," *Soc Psychiatry Psychiatr Epidemiol*, no. 39 (2004):797–803.

2   P. S. Appelbaum, "Almost a Revolution: An International Perspective on the Law of Involuntary Commitment," *Am Acad Psychiatry Law*, no. 25 (1997):135–47.

3   Xin C. Y., *Interpretation of the Mental Health Law of the People's Republic of China* (Beijing: China Legal Publishing House, 2012), 356.

ment, i.e., the demand principle.[1] During that time, however, a complex mix of factors emerged, including opposition to psychiatry and the civil rights movement[2] and permission for more effective treatments, such as community treatment. As a result, the civil commitment attracted the attention of the public and the legislature, and problems seemed to arise in what had previously been a seemingly beneficial approach.[3]

The dangerousness principle was codified in the laws of the District of Columbia and California in 1964 and 1969, respectively.[4] However, the widespread adoption of the dangerousness principle in the United States originated from the Supreme Court's decision in O'Connor v. Donaldson.[5] It was later argued that such measures against people who were not at risk were unconstitutional, despite not being the intention of the courts.[6] The dangerousness principle is generally expressed as a substantial likelihood of imminent harm to others or oneself as a result of mental illness. In layman's terms, it means that there is a "risk of harm to oneself or others."[7] Compulsory medical treatment is only permitted if the failure to treat the mentally disordered person poses a danger to the mentally disordered person and others, or known as the dangerousness principle. "Dangerousness" has long been used by legislators to justify intervention in the freedoms of the mentally disordered and the use of police powers by governments. The dangerousness principle was applied in various countries before the nineteenth century. However, it was more often provided for in administrative

---

1   T. Szasz, "Commitment of the Mentally Ill: Treatment or Social Straint," *J Nerv Ment Dis*, no. 125 (1957): 293–307.

2   A. A. Stone, *Mental Health and Law: A System in Transition* (Washington D. C.: National Institute of Mental Health, 1975).

3   R. R. Parlour, "The Reorganisation of the California Department of Mental Hygiene," *Am J Psychiatry*, no. 128 (1972):1388–1394.

4   A. H. Urmer, "Implications of California's New Mental Health Law," *Am J Psychiatry*, no. 132 (1975): 251-254.

5   O'Connor v. Donaldson, 422US563.1975.

6   S. A. Anfang, "Appelbaum PS. Civil Commitment: The American Experience," *Isr J Psychiatry Relat Sci*, no. 43 (2006): 209-218.

7   Bruce J. Cohen, Richard J. Bonnie, and John Monahan, "Understanding and Applying Virginia's New Statutory Civil Commitment Criteria," *Developments in Mental Health Law* (July 2009): 132.

decrees or state policies and was characterized as a "measure of security." With the enactment of mental health laws in various places and the development of the international human rights movement, the dangerousness principle has become more widely applied in areas of public law.[1]

II. Standard of Compulsory Medical Treatment for Mental Disorders Established by the Mental Health Law: Dangerousness Principle

Article 30 of the Mental Health Law of the People's Republic of China sets out the standards for compulsory medical treatment of persons with mental disorders in China: first of all, diagnostic conclusions and assessment of the patient's condition indicate that the patient is suffering from a serious mental disorder. The Mental Health Law specifies that the patients who are first institutionalized must have evidence of suffering from certain severe mental disorders, i.e., the six categories of mental disorders (schizophrenia, schizoaffective disorder, paranoid psychosis, bipolar affective disorder, epilepsy-induced mental disorders, mental retardation) as defined by the Regulations on the Management and Treatment of Serious Mental Illnesses (Ministry of Health, 2012). Involuntary hospitalization is possible only for persons with severe mental disorders who meet specific criteria. The principle of voluntary hospitalization is applied to patients with general mental disorders.

Secondly, the patient must have committed an act that harms him/herself or poses a risk of harm to him/herself or has committed an act that jeopardizes the safety of others. In the first case, the patient must have committed an act or risk of harm to himself/herself or have committed an act or risk of harm to the safety of others. In this case, the patient's condition is so serious that the patient has already done harm to him or herself or is at risk of doing so. If he or she is not hospitalized, he or she will suffer even

---

1 Zhang W. T., "Study on the Civilian Commitment System for the People with Mental Illness," Shandong University, 2011.

more serious consequences of harming himself or herself. For this reason, it is necessary to hospitalize the patient in order to protect his/her life and health. The second situation is when the patient has already committed an act that endangers the safety of others or is at risk of endangering the safety of others. In this case, the person with a severe mental disorder has already endangered the safety of others and has caused harmful consequences or is at risk of doing so. Failure to hospitalize the patient will result in more serious consequences for the personal and property safety of others. Therefore, it is necessary to hospitalize the patient in order to prevent further deterioration of the patient's condition and safeguard the safety of others. A patient who suffers from either of the above two conditions is eligible for involuntary hospitalization under the Mental Health Law.

It is clear that the standard for hospitalization under the Mental Health Law of the People's Republic of China is the dangerousness principle. Special attention should be paid to the fact that the dangerousness principle is likely to be implemented with the risk of being arbitrarily amplified. The terms "harming oneself" and "endangering the safety of others" in Article 30 of the Mental Health Law of the People's Republic of China should be interpreted as "threat to life" or "possibility of serious bodily harm." Minor physical or emotional harm should be excluded. Danger, in this context, refers to the imminent risk of death,[1] as exemplified by suicides and violent assaults. Moreover, such "harm" or "danger" should be highly "probable" and clearly "imminent." Patients with mental disorders should not be compulsorily committed if they present only a mere verbal threat, with no substantial preparatory behavior for "harm" or "endangerment." If the mentally disordered person only exhibits mental disturbances to him or herself or others, such as begging or wandering in the street, with no visible danger, other alternative measures (such as outpatient treatment or medication) should be taken rather than simply applying compulsory medical treatment such as restricting personal liberty.

The mainstream view on determining whether the behavior of a patient with mental disorders is "dangerous" is based on the following five aspects:

---

1   J. Hewitt, "Dangerousness and Mental Health Policy," *Journal of Psychiatric and Mental Health Nursing* 151, no. 3 (2008): 86–94.

(1) the type of conduct (physical assault, threat of conduct, verbal threat, property damage, purposeless injury); (2) the frequency of the conduct; (3) the frequency of the conduct (number of days prior to filing); (4) the method of injury (what instrument); and (5) the object of the conduct (other, self, or both).[1] Appelbaum adds the person's personal factors to the dangerousness principle, such as a patient's impaired capacity to act,[2] which is of great importance in practice.

III. Dangerousness Principle Derived from an Unfair Assessment of Risk

The inclusion of the dangerousness principle in the Mental Health Act relies on the assumption that a person with a mental illness can be reliably assessed by a medical professional as to whether he or she is at risk of harm.[3] It is usually argued that there is sufficient evidence to ensure the reliability of the diagnosis of serious mental illness. However, scholars, including Large and Ryan, believe that there is no reliable approach to assessing the risk of harm.[4]

Way and his colleagues assessed patients with mental disorders brought to the emergency room on the basis of video recordings and examined the reliability of the assessments among senior emergency psychiatrists. Although they found a high degree of agreement in the diagnosis of mental disorders, there was only a low level of reliability in assessing the risk of patients posing a danger to themselves and others.[5]

---

1   Virginia Aldige Hiday, "Court Discretion: Application of the Dangerousness Standard in Civil Commitment," *Law and Human Behavior* 5. no. 4 (1981): 278.

2   P. Appelbaum, "Almost a Revolution: An International Perspective on the Law of Involuntary Commitment," *The Journal of the American Academy of Psychiatry and the Law*, no. 25 (1997):135–147.

3   M. D. Warner and C. A. Peabody, "Reliability of Diagnoses Made by Psychiatric Residents in a General Emergency Department," *Psychiatr Serv.*, no. 46 (1995):1284–1286.

4   M. M. Large, C. J. Ryan, O. B. Nielssen, and R. A. Hayes, "The Danger of Dangerousness," *Law, Ethics, and Medicine*, no. 34 (2008): 877–881.

5   B. B. Way et al., "Inter Agreement among Psychiatrists in Psychiatric Emergency Assessments," *Am J Psychiatry*, no. 155 (1998): 1423–1428.

To examine the risk of violence more directly, the MacArthur Research Group on Mental Illness and Violence determined the risk of violence for patients discharged from hospitals using constructed interviews.[1] They tested actuarial modeling in a second cohort.[2] This study showed that patients in the low-risk group had a nine times higher risk of violence than the expected 1%, while those in the high-risk group committed 45% less violence than expected. Although the sensitivity and specificity of Monahan's calculations were only 70% and 72%, respectively, 29% of the patients were misclassified. The results would be even more disappointing if the model for predicting the risk of violence were used on a group of hospitalized patients. The discharged patients in the Monahan study had a high rate of risky violence. Eighteen percent of all patients and 35% of high-risk patients were found to behave violently during the follow-up visit. Given that hospitalized patients tend to have a low base rate of violence, signal monitoring theory indicates that the predictive reliability of a risk is much lower.[3] If it is used for patients being considered for hospitalization, more of them will be misclassified by this approach. Therefore, this tool for predicting risky violence is supposed to have the best evidence base, but it is of limited utility.

Scholars have found that the original intention of using assessment tools to predict who is at risk of suicide has not been fulfilled.[4] Pokorny describes an influential prospective trial that predicted suicide risks for patients based on their condition at the time of hospitalization.[5] Despite extensive and repeated data review, scholars did not detect any clinical utility in the combination of clinical symptoms and other factors.[6] A few studies then attempted

---

1   J. Monahan, H. Steadman, and E. Silver, *Rethinking Risk Assessment: The MacArthur Study of Mental Disorder and Violence* (Oxford: Oxford University Press, 2001).

2   J. Monahan et al., "An Actuarial Model of Violence Risk Assessment for Persons with Mental Disorders," *Psychiatr Serv.*, no. 56 (2005): 810–815.

3   D. Mossman and E. Somoza, "Neuropsychiatric Decision Making: The Role of Disorder Prevalence in Diagnostic Testing," *Neuropsychiatry Clin Neurosci*, no. 3 (1991): 84–88.

4   A. D. Pokorny., "Prediction of Suicide in Psychiatric Patients: Report of a Prospective Study," *Arch Gen Psychiatry*, no. 40 (1983): 249–257.

5   Ibid., "Suicide Prediction Revisited," *Suicide Life Threat Behav.*, no. 23 (1993): 1-10.

6   I. M. Hunt et al., "Suicide in Current Psychiatric In-Patients: A Case-Control Study," *Psychol Med.*, no. 37 (2007): 831–837.

to predict the risk of suicide. The exception was studies that attempted to examine predictive signals of suicide in hospitalized patients. But even in these studies, those who tried to commit suicide had the same demographic and clinical characteristics as those who did not try to commit suicide. In addition, suicide commonly occurs during periods of low risk.[1]

These studies emphasize that physicians know that, even under ideal circumstances, psychiatrists cannot accurately or precisely predict a patient's risk of harming themselves or others. In practice, it would imply that if it is common in reality that involuntary hospitalization decisions are made on the basis of risk prediction, psychiatrists have made safety errors. Many individuals are kept in hospital ostensibly because of possible future risks, but they may never become dangerous.

IV. Legal Discrimination in the Dangerousness Principle

There seems to be nothing wrong with compulsory medical treatment of patients with mental disorders who may cause harm to themselves or others. However, is this true? If it is considered reasonable, why do legislators and stakeholders in Europe and the United States argue for a long time without coming to an acceptable conclusion? Currently, there is a relatively common consensus in mental health legislation in various countries on compulsory medical treatment for patients with mental disorders, also known as the dangerousness principle. Is this principle correct? Is there any discrimination in applying the dangerousness principle to compulsory medical treatment of patients with mental disorders?

Assuming that two persons, A and B, have a serious tendency to violence, A is not mentally disordered and has been sent to prison for his sentence. Although he is still a danger to others, he will be released at the end of his sentence. B suffers from a severe mental disorder (assuming bipolar affective disorder) and is committed to a closed mental hospital. He

---

1   Dong J. Y., Ho T. P., and Kan C. K., "A Case-Control Study of 92 Cases of In-Patient Suicides," *Affect Disord.*, no. 87 (2005): 91–99.

will remain in the hospital as long as he is recognized as a danger to others. It follows that two persons who are both dangerous: one with a mental disorder is confined indefinitely in a closed hospital to prevent any harm to others, while the other, who does not have a mental disorder, is released at the end of his term of imprisonment.

What exactly justifies A's freedom after serving his sentence, while B, who suffers from a mental disorder, is subjected to indefinite mandatory imprisonment? If the only reason for imprisoning B is that he is still a danger to others, A should continue to be imprisoned. But it is against the law to imprison A after A has served a full sentence. Perhaps it is simpler to make a risk assessment of A and B, and perhaps the risk factor is higher for persons with mental disorders who have a record of violent acts. But suppose that these facts, if they can be counted at all, provide a basis for detaining patients with mental disorders indefinitely. Would it be reasonable to detain a person with mental capacity if he or she presented the same degree of foreseeable danger as a person with a mental disorder? A more plausible reason for detaining B indefinitely would be that he might consent to his own incarceration while he remains a danger to others. However, this rationale may not be sufficient to explain similar cases. In the final analysis, B did not necessarily consent to his imprisonment.

It might be argued that the frequency and predicted capacity of Patient B's violent behavior make patients with mental disorders subject to special treatment. But is the risk of violent behavior only prevalent in people with mental disorders? In fact, most violent acts are committed by people without mental disorders, and no evidence suggests that violent behavior is more predictable in people with mental disorders than in those without (e.g., those who engage in domestic violence and heavy drinking).[1] Even if violent behavior is proven in people with mental disorders, why should they be forced to accept preventive restrictions when those who engage in domestic violence and heavy drinking are not forced to accept preventive measures?

---

1   H. Steadman et al., "Violence by People Discharged from Acute Psychiatric Inpatient Facilities and by Others in the Same Neighborhoods," *Arch Gen Psychiatry* 55, no. 5 (May 1998): 393–401.

The system of criminal sanctions in democratic countries provides a good example of our common methods, which are applied in a completely opposite way. Those accused of violent crimes are supposed to be innocent until proven guilty. "It is better for ten guilty persons to escape than for one innocent person to be convicted."[1] Few laws allow for the imprisonment of innocent persons, even when they are recognized to be at risk of harming others in the future.

Even more ridiculously, the dangerousness principle usually excludes personality disorders from the scope of compulsory medical treatment. Even the Mental Health Law of the People's Republic of China excludes personality disorders from the six categories of severe mental disorders. This is mainly because there are no effective therapies or treatments for patients with personality disorders. However, personality disorders are actually among the many mental disorders that are likely to pose a danger to society. In particular, DSPD (Dangerous and Severe Personality Disorder) refers to those with antisocial personality disorders (narrowly defined as psychopathic personality) and records of violent acts. As a result, it is proposed to minimize the risks posed by these individuals. Section 4 of the British Mental Health Act 1983 defines such mental disorders as "a persistent psychological disorder or loss of functioning (with or without subnormal intelligence) which often leads to the development of abnormally aggressive or seriously irresponsible acts in some patients." Starting with this definition, it complements the conventional description of the possibility that personality disorders lead only to the patient's self-suffering. As a result, the coverage of personality diagnosis has been broadened.[2] On the contrary, "dangerous and severe personality disorders" are excluded from the scope of compulsory medical treatment, which explicitly contradicts the purpose of compulsory medical treatment.[3]

---

1   W. Blackstone, *Commentaries on the Laws of England.* bk. 4 (1809), 27.

2   M. Gelder, P. Harrison, and P. Cowen, eds., *Shorter Oxford Textbook of Psychiatry*, 5th ed., trans. Liu X. H. and Li T. (Sichuan: Sichuan University Press, 2010), 146.

3   J. Bindman, S. Maingay, and G. Szmukler, "The Human Rights Act and Mental Health Legislation," *Br J Psychiatry*, no. 182 (2003): 91–94.

V. Dangerousness Principle Not Necessitated by Compulsory Medical Treatment

It is generally accepted in democratic countries that everyone can do what-ever they want as long as they do not cause harm to others. When the Mental Health Law was drafted, legislators commonly argued that provisions allow-ing treatment of uninformed patients with mental disorders implied a lim-itation on their autonomy. They wanted to incorporate the dangerousness principle into the law because they believed that a valid reason was needed for interfering with patients' autonomy. After all, they thought that everyone should be able to do whatever they wanted as long as they did not cause harm to others. If that is what the legislators want, their ideas are flawed.

In many cases, patients with mental disorders refuse psychiatric treat-ments because their mental disorders deprive them of the "capacity to consent to treatment." They have not made a deliberate decision to refuse treatment, nor can they do so. In many cases of refusal, the mental disorder deprives the patient of the capacity to be aware of their illness, how it affects them, and the benefits they would receive from treatment. If patients do not have the capacity to consent to treatment, they cannot be considered to have exercised their autonomy by refusing treatment. As a result, mental health laws, which provide for the compulsory treatment of patients with mental disorders who are unable to make decisions independently, do not violate the autonomy of these individuals. Their autonomy has been stripped away by their mental illness. Since their autonomy is not further diminished, there is no need to justify the legal neglect of autonomy. Nor is there a need to make the dangerousness principle a valid ground for defense.

Mental illness does not always deprive the patient of the decision to re-ceive treatment or the capacity to refuse medical treatment. When patients with mental disorders remain capable of making treatment decisions, they will mostly agree to some form of treatment because they can tell that it is in their best interest to do so. There are also very few examples. That is, pa-tients with mental disorders who can still make treatment decisions some-times refuse treatment even though they would benefit from it. A patient's capacity to refuse treatment is rarely considered an ethical issue unless the refusal of treatment poses a severe danger to others. How should the law deal with those rare situations where the risks associated with the capacity to refuse exceed the prescribed limits? Such a refusal may be similar to the case where a person with epilepsy refuses antiepileptic medication, and his or her condition progresses. It stands to reason that the dangers associated with the capacity of refusing should be dealt with under criminal law, instead of being subjected to compulsory medical treatment.

It is also noteworthy that the dangerousness principle can lead to the stigmatization of patients with mental disorders. As a result, these patients become more and more resistant to the services of psychiatrists, which is ultimately not conducive to long-term mental health prevention and treatment. The dangerousness principle may intensify social and public prejudice and discrimination against people with mental illness. Link et al. found from interviews that the percentage of the population perceiving people with mental illness as "dangerous" had actually increased from 4.2% in 1950 to 44.0% in 1996. They suggested that a possible reason for this was the widespread adoption of the dangerousness principle in the United States. It objectively popularizes and reinforces the view that mental illness is as dangerous as violent assault.[1]

VI. Dangerousness Principle with More Potential Disadvantages than Advantages

The dangerousness principle may cause harm to many patients with mental disorders and increase the risk of social harm. Legislators have chosen to apply the dangerousness principle because they see it as a legal justification for neglecting patients' autonomy. Another potential reason is that many people simply assume that the dangerousness principle protects patients with mental disorders and the community from harm. These views are completely wrong. New evidence highlighting First Episode Psychosis (FEP) suggests that the dangerousness principle may increase the risk of mental

---

1 B. G. Link, J. C. Phelan, M. Bresnahan, A. Stueve, and B. A. Pescosolido, "Public Conceptions of Mental Illness: Labels, Causes, Dangerousness, and Social Distance," *Am J Public Health* 89, no. 9 (1999): 1328–1333.

illness harming patients and substantially worsening dangers in the community.

As we discussed above, studies in the 1870s and early 1880s, when the dangerousness principle was first implemented, failed to identify any definitive and consistent adverse effects of the new law. Any fear of harm from the new law was considered anachronistic. Although people with mental disorders are often viewed as a separate group in these studies, no one has categorized patients with FEP separately. It was not until after 1980 that the concept of the FEP was presented in the literature. According to Large, patients with FEP represent only a small proportion of all patients with mental disorders, but they are largely unlike previously treated patients. New evidence suggests that the development of the dangerousness principle may have a detrimental effect on the course of FEP.[1]

Duration of Untreated Psychosis (DUP) refers to the period from the onset of symptoms of a mental illness to the time when appropriate treatment is administered.[2] In a recent study, Large compared the DUP of schizophrenia-related disorders with and without the dangerousness principle in studies from developed Western countries. Patients residing in jurisdictions with the dangerousness principle were delayed in initiating treatment by five months compared to those without the dangerousness principle.[3] This delay cannot be attributed to differences in patients' clinical characteristics, nor can it be explained by health service inputs. Rather, the presence of the dangerousness principle induces prolongation of the DUP in patients with FEP.

Delayed treatment is detrimental to patients with FEP. Two recent systematic evaluation projects investigated the vast amount of recent literature on delays in the initial phase of treatment for people with psychiatric disorders. They similarly concluded that prolonged DUPs have adverse effects on patients in clinical, psychosocial, and social aspects. A prolonged DUP

---

1   M. M. Large, C. J. Ryan, O. B Nielssen, R A Hayes. "The Danger of Dangerousness," *Law, Ethics, and Medicine*, no. 34 (2008,): 877–881.

2   R. M. Norman and A. K. Malla, "Duration of Untreated Psychosis: A Critical Examination of the Concept and Its Importance," *Psychol Med.*, no. 31 (2001): 381–400.

3   M. Large et al., "Mental Health Acts That Require Dangerousness for Involuntary Admission May Delay the Initial Treatment of Schizophrenia," *Soc Psychiatry Psychiatr Epidemiol*, no. 43 (2008): 251–256.

may also lead to an increase in suicidal behavior. Contrary to the findings of research conducted 30 years ago, the new evidence suggests that the dangerousness principle may have a detrimental effect on people in the early stages of mental illness.[1]

The negative effects of the dangerousness principle are not limited to mental illness. It is well documented that patients are at high risk of being violent toward others during FEP, and many studies have demonstrated that prolonged DUP is associated with an increase in violent behaviors. Unreasonably, clinicians always assess the likelihood of patients being violent based on their past record of violent acts. Patients in FEP merely had no time to act violently in the past, and therefore, they are not considered to be at serious risk for violence. If the risk of harm to the patients themselves or others is the primary reason for deciding to treat a non-consenting patient, it is reasonable to believe that patients in FEP are likely to be misclassified depending on the risk of harm, simply because of the short duration of their condition.[2]

VII. Seeking Alternative Standards to the Dangerousness Principle

1. Alternative criteria proposed by Large

Large argues that mental health legislators should reset the criteria and conditions for compulsory medical treatment of patients: (1) Independent assessors believe that patients with mental disorders lack the capacity to consent to certain treatments. (2) Independent assessors believe that patients with mental disorders would receive significant benefit from the

---

1 D. O. Perkins et al., "Relationship between Duration of Untreated Psychosis and Outcome in First-Episode Schizophrenia: A Critical Review and Meta-Analysis," *Am J Psychiatry*, no. 162 (2005): 1785–1804.

2 I. Melle et al., "Early Detection of the First Episode of Schizophrenia and Suicidal Behavior," *Am J Psychiatry*, no. 163 (2006): 800–804.

proposed treatment, or the proxy decision-maker believes that the patient would consent to the treatment if the patient had the capacity to make the decision. (3) Treatment should be delivered in the least restrictive environment and be highly practical.[1] This standard bears some resemblance to the legal model proposed by the American Psychiatric Association more than 20 years ago, returning the fulcrum of compulsory medical treatment to its original position.[2]

Clinicians should still make some estimate of a patient's potential for dangerous behavior. Despite its possible shortcomings, it will not be the core that governs compulsory medical treatment. Risk assessment only affects the decision on Criterion 3 and the availability of a treatment setting that is appropriate for the patient. If the new criteria are applied, the DUP for patients in FEP will be shortened, and they will receive more immediate treatment. Whether or not patients with mental disorders receive compulsory medical treatment will be determined by their capacity of conduct rather than by divining their future dangerousness.

2. Substitute standards proposed by Richardson

Concerns about patient autonomy can be traced back at least to 1999, when a section of the Richardson-led Committee of Experts published comments on the Mental Health Act. The Committee's report raised the question of whether we should respect the autonomy of a patient with mental disorders in the same way that we respect the autonomy of a patient with a physical illness. Patients with physical illnesses may refuse treatment out of their own will. However, in the case of patients with mental disorders, the Mental Health Act allows physicians to impose compulsory treatment, even if the patients retain the capacity to make a decision.[3] The Committee of Experts then established two basic principles that mental health legislation

---

1   M. M. Large, C. J. Ryan, O. B. Nielssen, and R. A. Hayes, "The Danger of Dangerousness," *Law, Ethics, and Medicine*, no. 34 (2008): 877–881.

2   C. D. Stromberg and A. A. Stone, "A Model State Law on Civil Commitment of the Mentally Ill," *Harvard J Legis.*, no. 20 (1983): 275–396.

3   Department of Health, "Review of the Mental Health Act 1983: Report of the Expert Committee," London: DoH, 1999.

must comply with: one is that persons with mental disorders should not be discriminated against and should be treated on an equal footing with persons suffering from other illnesses. The second is to respect their autonomy. These two principles have led to a rethinking of compulsory medical treatment, and it has been concluded that compulsory medical treatment must be determined as a result of a patient's lack of capacity. Capacity refers to the ability of the patient to understand the nature and purpose of the recommended treatment, including the consequences of having or not having received the treatment, before making a decision. Szmukler also agrees with the Committee's views on "capacity." Capacity must be the priority of mental health law, whereas an unspecified definition of "mental disorder" is secondary to the decisions about involuntary treatment.[1] The two most important points are whether the patient has the capacity to decide on his or her choice of treatment and, assuming that the patient has the capacity to decide, whether the treatment of the patient is in the patient's best interests. The Committee is therefore able to accept a broad definition of mental disorders. "Capacity" also forces us to ascertain whether the true purpose of treatment is "for the health and safety of the patient" or "for the protection of others." In Scotland, the Mental Health Act 2003 stipulates that the "loss of decision-making capacity" of patients with mental disorders is one of the central criteria for physicians to impose compulsory medical treatment. Thus, it also sets a precedent for us to follow the Act.[2]

3. Supplementing the evidence on "capacity of refusing medical treatment" as an evaluation criterion

Mental health legislation in some US states (most of which still apply the dangerousness principle today) and Scotland states that the assessment of the "capacity of refusing medical treatment" should be supplemented on the basis of the dangerousness principle as a criterion for compulsory medical treatment of patients with mental disorders.

---

1   George Szmukler and Frank Holloway, "Reform of the Mental Health Act: Health or Safety?," *BJP*, no. 177 (2000): 196–200.

2   Mental Health (Care and Treatment) (Scotland) Act 2003. Clause 57(3) (d).

The criteria for compulsory institutionalization under the Mental Health Act for Scotland (2003) are based on a comprehensive assessment and decision-making in the following five conditions:[1] Firstly, "mental disorder" means that the patient must have an objective mental disorder. Secondly, it must be "treatable," implying that it must provide possible medical treatment: (1) to prevent the mental disorder from worsening and (2) to alleviate the patient's symptoms, reactions, or disorders by means adapted to the patient. Treatment here is considered to be broad, encompassing medication and specific psychotherapeutic treatments, as well as nursing care, support, specialized therapies, and social rehabilitation measures. Although clinically refractory schizophrenia may appear to be untreatable, there is much that can be done in practice to mitigate or prevent the deterioration of the patient's condition. Thirdly, the patient's condition must be dangerous, meaning that the patient would be at great risk if he or she did not receive such medical treatment: (1) The patient's health, safety, and well-being should be guaranteed. (2) The safety of any other person should be guaranteed. It is important to note that the danger test here is set at a low threshold and involves participants who have a propensity for violence against themselves and others. Danger involves the health or well-being of the person. Risks may include, for example, self-neglect, inability to manage finances appropriately, serious damage to human relationships, or inability to care for children. But whatever the risk is, it must be caused by a direct or indirect mental disorder. Fourthly, the patient must have a lack of capacity (or "capacity of refusing medical treatment"), i.e., the patient is unable to make a decision as to whether he or she needs such medical treatment because of his or her mental disorder. Special attention should be paid here to the fact that the capacity test is innovative. Capacity is the ability to make decisions about mental treatment. Patients with impaired decision-making capacity have lower thresholds than those without capacity. In practice, it needs to be considered that a patient with a mental disorder (e.g., delusional disorders, lack of cognitive capacity, lack of insight) has a disorder that may affect the person's decision-making capacity and influence the mental treatment given to the person. Consideration must be given to

---

1   Rajan Darjee, "The Mental Health Act in Scotland," *Professional Skills* (2008): 20.

the impact of mental disorders on a person's capacity for understanding. It is important to ascertain, retain, and weigh relevant information in order to reach a reasoned decision. A patient who does not consent to treatment by a physician does not mean that he or she does not need treatment. Finally, compulsory medical treatment should be imperative, meaning that it is necessary to apply it to patients and that it cannot be replaced by any other means.

History of the Protection of the Rights of Patients with Mental Disorders in the United States and Implications

I. History and Development of Protecting the Rights of Patients with Mental Disorders in the United States

1. Early history of protecting the rights of patients with mental disorders in the United States

During the colonial period in the United States, there was no standardized accreditation of patients with mental diseases and their treatment and entitlement services. In fact, at that time, many patients with mental disorders were deemed to have been bewitched by witches or to be witches themselves and would be turned over to the church for trial and punishment. Soon afterward, patients with mental disorders were no longer banished or deported to small huts on the edge of farms or to neighboring towns. Instead, they were delivered by township officials to a series of large institutions funded and operated by the county: almshouses (for ruffians and hoodlums), poorhouses (for the poor and widows, etc.), and reformatories (for drunkards and troublemakers). In practice, people with mental disorders stayed in these institutions for longer periods and were considered to be incarcerated to some extent.[1]

2. Development of the protection of the rights of patients with mental disorders in the United States

In 1776, 13 states adopted the US Constitution and the United States Bill of Rights and called on all US citizens to adopt and exercise the rights protected in the bill. These rights included the right to practice religion, the right to freedom of speech, the right to freedom of the press, the right to peaceful assembly, the right to bring public grievances to the government's attention, and the right to keep and bear arms. An overview of the United States Bill of Rights reveals that the vast majority of its provisions deal with legal procedures, and only a very small percentage, even indirectly, can be applied to patients with mental disorders. However, it must be pointed out that patients with mental disorders are generally and customarily considered ineligible for these rights.

During that period, reformers worked to improve the care of patients with mental disorders in a variety of institutions. Among these reformers, the most famous was a woman named Dorothea Dix, who argued in the 1840s that patients with mental disorders should be hospitalized in federally funded hospitals, away from the pressures of the big cities and county institutions with shocking residential and mental health problems. This plan for the federal government to assume responsibility for the medical care of patients with mental disorders never materialized. However, the states did assume this responsibility, establishing a network of hundreds of state hospitals in all 50 states in time. Situated in quiet, idyllic neighborhoods, these hospitals did their best to provide patients with attentive and friendly nursing staff and allowed these patients to dine in a room that looked like their own dining room. However, because patients could not leave the hospitals at will, these hospitals became overcrowded as immigrants flooded the

---

1   J. A. Talbott, "Managed Care in France: How What's Happened in America Can Sweep France Unless You Understand Why It Happened and Change," *L'Evolution Psychiatrique*, no. 64 (1999): 495–510.

coasts of the United States. These hospitals were more like warehouses than hospitals. The most significant milestones in the history of the protection of the rights of patients with mental disorders in the United States occurred in 1867 and 1874.

> ### The right of the jury to hear civil suits against hospitals (1867)

Despite efforts to provide humane, caring, and open services, mental hospitals (state psychiatric hospitals) failed to do so, and abuses of civil commitment occasionally occurred. In 1867, Elizabeth Packard, a patient treated at the Illinois State Hospital for Mental Diseases, pushed the legislature to pass a law requiring all involuntary psychiatric treatments to be subject to the trial and approval of a jury. Since that time, the states have gradually introduced relevant legal review procedures. They require that patients in practical need of compulsory medical treatment be examined and diagnosed by a physician who is not affiliated with the hospital before they can be admitted. Patients with mental disorders then are entitled to request a judicial hearing within a specified number of days. Although each state has separate laws and procedures, there are universal and comprehensive standards for the procedures necessary to compel civil commitment to medical treatment.[1] This system of judicial hearings was first applied to patients who could be improved by treatment or who had become a danger to themselves or others. However, the standards have become more stringent. In some cases, a person can only be involuntarily institutionalized if he or she poses a threat to others with a gun in his or her hand or is unable to care for himself or herself outside of a medical facility in the state. These legal processes and procedures may become cumbersome and obstructive for these patients.[2] It is worth noting that many states have long been implementing "conditional releases," which require patients with mental disorders to be readmitted to the hospital if they experience a deterioration in their condition after being discharged from the hospital.

---

1   M. S. Himmelhoch and A. H. Shaffer, "Elizabeth Packard: Nineteenth Century Crusader for the Rights of Mental Patients," *Am Stud.*, no. 13 (1979): 343–375.

2   P. S. Appelbaum, "Civil Mental Health Law: Twenty Years of History and a Look at the Future," *Mental and Physical Disability LawReporter*, no. 20 (1996): 599–604.

> ### *Patient's Bill of Rights (1874)*

The United States is a multi-state union. The 50 states have supreme authority over the federal government in many ways. And each state's sphere of
influence, whether in terms of laws, regulations, or procedures, has been
separated from the rest of the country for as long as history has lasted. It
means that in one area, such as the rights and interests of patients with mental disorders, each state has its statutes, regulations, and rules. Thus, while
one state's laws or lawsuits may affect other areas of the country, other states
are not obligated to do the same. As a supplement to the United States Bill of
Rights, the earliest statute laws addressing patients' interests and rights can
be traced back to the 18th century. As early as 1874 and 1879, the Commonwealth of Massachusetts enacted laws clarifying patients' rights to correspondence and visitation. In 1947, 1948, and 1951, Vermont, Michigan, and
Illinois provided for the right of patients to be visited by their defense attorneys, the right of patients to receive proper care, attention, and treatment,
and the right of agencies to intervene in investigations of cruel, negligent, or
inappropriate treatment of patients.

A milestone in the protection of patients' rights was the 1971 case of
Wyatt v. Stickney. It was only then that states began to define patients' rights
and set standards in a more detailed and precise manner. These state governments stipulate that patients shall have the right to receive appropriate
treatment and services, the right to an individualized therapeutic regimen
and to periodic review of the program for modification, and the right to
a plan of care after treatment of the disease. In addition, patients may be
entitled to the right to be treated in a humane environment, the right to privacy and security, the right to refuse treatment, the right to speak in private,
and the right to explain the therapeutic regimen. They also have the right to
access their treatment records, the right to information about their rights,
the right to address their grievances, and the right to make a legal statement
and/or secure a defense attorney. Additionally, they have the right to the
civil rights available to all citizens: the right to freedom of religion, the right
to be paid for their work, the right to vote, the right to physical exercise and
outdoor recreation, the right to a nutritious diet, and the right to be visited
by a person of the opposite sex. In 1975, the District of Columbia and the
State of Montana emphasized the rights of patients with mental disorders to

be released from hospitals and to receive post-discharge care, and the right to be free from discrimination in their residences.

II. Content of the Protection of the Rights of Patients with Mental Disorders in the United States

1. The right of patients with mental disorders to correspondence and visitation (1874)

The Commonwealth of Massachusetts considered the rights of patients with mental disorders to correspondence and visitation as early as 1874, but not all states followed suit. Weiner documented that 45 states had enacted laws that guaranteed patients' communication with the outside world, 38 states had enacted laws allowing telephone calls, and 47 states had enacted statute laws guaranteeing the right of patients to communicate with the outside world via mail.[1]

2. The right to informed consent for patients with mental disorders (1914)

It is the right of all patients (initially limited to patients with medical treatments) in the United States. In other words, no medical practice is allowed to be imposed on anyone. Whereas before, it was only considered a due, now it has become defined as a right to be decided by a court. In 1914, every sane adult was entitled to decide which treatments he or she would receive for his or her body. If a patient was operated on without consent, the act was deemed a crime, and the physician would be held liable for damages. In 1972, this regulation was further refined to include the right of the patient

---

1   B. A. Weiner, "Provider-Patient Relations: Confidentiality and Liability," chap. 10 of *The Mentally Disabled and the Law*, ed. S. J. Brakel, J. Parry, and B. A. Weiner, 3rd ed. (Chicago: American Bar Foundation, 1985), 559–605.

to know his or her diagnosis, the nature and risks of treatment, the expected consequences of withholding treatment, and alternative treatments.[1]

3. The right of patients with mental disorders to receive medical treatment (1960)

Birnbaum recommended that patients in facilities for the treatment of mental diseases have the right to be treated; otherwise, they are no different from being imprisoned.[2] In the 1966 case of Rouse v. Cameron, Judge David Bazelon held that indefinite delay in treatment was a cruel and unusual punishment for a patient with mental disorders who had not committed a crime. It was consistent with the Eighth Amendment to the Constitution of the United States. The judge authored a resolution that would later have great influence: "Medical institutions were established for the purpose of healing, not punishing." It was in 1972, in the case of Wyatt v. Stickney, that specific standards for adequate medical treatment were actually set, including the setting, the medical personnel, and the treatment design. In 1974, another amendment to the Constitution led to another famous case, Donaldson v. O'Connor, which clarified that the right to be treated is constitutional. Currently, all states in the United States recognize the right to treatment.

4. The right of patients with mental disorders to receive remuneration for their labor in mental hospitals (1966)

In 1966, the federal government first adopted the Fair Labor Standards Act. In the mental hospitals of the 17th and 18th centuries, labor was considered a primary function of these hospitals. Patients with mental disorders who engaged in labor (e.g., on farms, in gardens, and in stores that made or repaired shoes and clothes) were considered to be in good condition and were receiving treatment. By the mid-20th century, however, side effects were be-

---

1 B. A. Weiner, "Treatment Rights," chap. 6 of *The Mentally Disabled and the Law*, ed. S. J. Brakel, J. Parry, and B. A. Weiner, 3rd ed. (Chicago: American Bar Foundation, 1985), 327–367

2 M. Birnbaum, "The Right to Treatment," *Am Bar Assoc J.*, no. 46 (1960): 499–505.

coming apparent. The New York State Psychiatric Hospital was exposed to a scandal when all the patients were building a yacht for the superintendent, because it was far more economical to hire unpaid patients with mental disorders to do the work than to hire workers at minimum wage.

It is evident that reforms were imperative. Unfortunately, the court's decision was intended to end "slave labor," but Souder points out that many of the reforms with good intentions have sadly ended up going astray. Many state hospitals were unwilling to adjust regulations, develop the necessary documents, involve projects that were supposed to be truly therapeutic, or pay patients with mental disorders for their labor.[1] As a result, by 1970, the wards had always been overcrowded.

5. The right to the minimum restriction in the treatment of patients with mental disorders (1966)

Since the introduction of the prescription drug phenothiazine in psychiatric hospitals in most states of the United States in 1955, patients with mental illness have been subjected to medical treatment even when they have been discharged from hospitals. It has also contributed to changes in attitudes (e.g., the belief that treatment in the community is better despite the absence of scientific evidence), economics (the fact that community healthcare is financed by the federal government), and the law. The change in the law has been pushed by a number of active and dedicated lawyers for rights protection, as well as by state organizations. Most of them were convinced that psychiatric hospitals were useless and that no treatment outside of institutions was better than treatment in those institutions, which were funded by the state. They advocated that treatment must take place in a minimally restrictive environment. This philosophy was first stated in 1966 by Judge Bazelon in the case of Lake v. Cameron: "People should not be treated in a restrictive environment (e.g., locked in a ward in a hospital), but in a more relaxing environment (e.g., a nursing home)." Although it was a good idea, some scholars have noted that the concept was gradually distorted into "any

---

1   Souder v. Brennan 367 F Supp. 808 (D. D. C. 1973).

place that would not be a state hospital."[1] In the 1970s, most lawyers sought such treatment for patients without real concern for those who needed it.

6. The right of patients with mental disorders to refuse treatment (1977)

A review indicated that about 10% of patients in the United States refused treatment, and about 20 to 25 % did not receive treatment.[2] Whether or not a patient has the right to refuse treatment remains a highly controversial issue among psychiatrists and lawyers. In the United States, people are accustomed to changing various areas and resolving most disagreements through legal processes. In litigation and legal disputes, many cases have been handled in an exaggerated manner. In the case of Davis v. Hubbard in 1980, for example, it was claimed that psychotropic drugs could be overprescribed and prescribed at will. Since 1977, many cases have protested the use of psychotropic drugs against the wishes of patients with mental disorders.

The history is long and complicated, but hospitals in every state in the US currently have mandated written procedures for administering psychotropic medications against a patient's wishes. If a group of physicians other than the attending team of a patient with mental disorders reviews and deems it necessary, or if a court deems it necessary to administer psychiatric medication against the patient's wishes, the medication may be administered in emergencies, for example, by signing a consent to receive the medication before the patient's condition worsens or the patient's seizure occurs.[3] In the United States, studies have shown that most patients are treated against their will in hospitals, but the results show that the treatment benefits them.[4] Neverthe-

---

1　M. R. Munetz and J. L. Geller, "The Least Restrictive Alternative in the Post-Institutional Era," *Hosp Community Psychiatry*, no. 44 (1993): 967–973.

2　P. S. Appelbaum, "Civil Mental Health Law: Twenty Years of History and a Look at the Future," *Mental and Physical Disability Law Reporter*, no. 20 (1996): 599–604.

3　Ibid., "Advance Directives for Psychiatric Care," *Hosp Community Psychiatry*, no. 42 (1991): 983–984.

4　H. I. Schwartz, W. Vingiano, and C. B. Perez, "Autonomy and the Right to Refuse Treatment: Patients' Attitudes after Involuntary Medication," *Hosp Community Psychiatry*, no. 39 (1988): 1049–1054.

less, these findings do not prevent people from questioning the dangerous-ness principle. The dangerousness principle means that patients with mental diseases can be treated without their consent once they are judged to have the potential to cause harm to themselves or others. Also, the dangerousness principle suggests that patients with mental disorders are subject to com-pulsory medical treatment without consent whenever they are considered to be at risk of harming themselves or others. However, the dangerousness principle has been called into question in recent years because, first of all, psychiatrists are not in a position to accurately assess the risk of harm to themselves or others for each patient. In practice, it implies that if the de-cision to involuntarily institutionalize a patient is based on a prediction of dangerousness, but the psychiatrist gets it wrong about safety (as is often the case), many patients who would otherwise be at little risk will be in-stitutionalized on the basis of such a false prediction. More importantly, the doctrine of criminal justice in the United States as a democracy teaches us the fundamental principle that those accused of violent crimes are pre-sumed innocent until proven guilty and that the state must prove their guilt beyond a mere shadow of a doubt. The principle of "in dubio pro reo" is one of the most fundamental principles in modern criminal law. Few pieces of legislation would allow the imprisonment of an innocent person simply because they have the potential to harm others in the future.[1]

Also, electro-convulsive therapy should not be overlooked. In the 1960s, electro-convulsive therapy became a major political issue. Scientologists in the United States consistently resisted its use. Although there is much sci-entific evidence of its effectiveness, hospitals and psychiatrists avoid its use, and electro-convulsive therapy is probably the effective approach that is still most sadly underused.

7. The right to freedom of religion and belief for patients with mental disorders (1979)

Although the right to freedom of religion was already guaranteed in the US Bill of Rights in 1776, many states have only recently found it necessary to

---

1   Wyatt v. Stickney, 325 F. Supp. 781, 784–85 (M.D. Ala 1971) (Johnson, CJ).

concretize this right in order to protect patients with mental disorders.[1] In 1985, half of the states in the United States had enacted provisions on the right to freedom of religion for patients with mental disorders.

8. The right of patients with mental disorders to work as internists (1982)

Current US law supports the right of some patients with mental disorders to work as internists. Once again, the courts have become a battleground for patients with mental disorders to fight for their rights, and the outcome is not yet known.[2]

9. The right of patients with mental disorders to smoke (1995)

Smoke-free areas have been established in the United States since 1980, but such areas have hardly been accessible to patients with mental disorders. State hospitals have adjusted their policies to allow patients with mental disorders who have been institutionalized for more than six months to smoke without a physician's permission. In fact, in some cases, physicians' permission and authorization have placed these physicians in a peculiar dilemma, both ethically and legally.

10. The right of patients with mental disorders to participate in elections

Although it is widely believed that patients with mental disorders cannot vote because they are incapable of making clear judgments, studies have shown that they are able to vote in the same way as the general population.

---

1   B. A. Weiner, "Rights of Institutionalized Persons," chap. 5 of *The Mentally Disabled and the Law*, ed. S. J. Brakel, J. Parry, and B. A. Weiner, 3rd ed. (Chicago: American Bar Foundation, 1985), 251–325.

2   P. S. Appelbaum, "Do the Mentally Disabled Have the Right to Be Physicians?," *Hosp Community Psychiatry*, no. 33 (1982): 351–352.

In 1976, all states except Louisiana allowed patients with mental disorders to cast absentee votes.[1]

11. The right of patients with mental disorders to privacy of communication

In the United States, a distinction is made between the privacy of communications between physicians and patients and the right to privacy. A physician cannot disclose any information about a patient with mental disorders without the patient's permission, except in the cases of child abuse or court order, or when the mental state of a patient with mental disorder constitutes part of a lawsuit. Such elements of patient privacy protections in interactions between physicians and patients have been legislated to varying degrees in different states. For example, in 1985, 34 states had laws protecting the privilege of privacy in physician-patient communications; 7 states had laws protecting the privacy of physicians and patients with mental diseases; 26 states had laws protecting the privacy of psychologists and patients; and 13 states had laws protecting the privacy of psychotherapists and patients. The scope of privacy protection here includes patients with mental disorders attempting to commit a crime or engaging in harmful behavior.

12. The right of patients with mental disorders to periodic review

As most practicing physicians know, the condition of patients with mental disorders is subject to change. In the United States, a study of 1,500 patients found significant changes in treatment plans and the level of treatment required. In addition to relying on mental health organizations, such reviews must be conducted regularly by experts independent of mental health organizations.

---

1   B. A. Weiner, "Rights of Institutionalized Persons," chap. 5 of *The Mentally Disabled and the Law*, ed. S. J. Brakel, J. Parry, and B. A. Weiner. 3rd ed. (Chicago: American Bar Foundation, 1985), 251–325.

III. Implications for China's Legislation on the Protection of the Rights of Patients with Mental Disorders in the United States

In recent years, some grassroots mental health workers in China have disregarded the rights and interests of people with mental illness, and have followed the conventional notions of the biomedical model, regarding involuntary institutionalization and treatment as an ordinary act of consumption. They are only responsible for the payer or the person who sends the patient for treatment and regard the payer as the object of their service while ignoring the basic rights of autonomy and self-determination of some patients who have the capacity to act. As a result, there have been many unimaginable and shocking cases of "being misdiagnosed with mental illness," such as the cases of Sun Fawu, He Jinrong, Zou Yijun, and Xu Lindong. In October 2011, the Twenty-Third Session of the Standing Committee of the Eleventh National People's Congress considered the Mental Health Law of the People's Republic of China (Draft) for the first time (hereinafter referred to as the Draft). The Draft has been openly solicited for comments from the public.[1] It should be considered progress, but the protection of the rights of people with mental disorders provided for in the Draft is rather disappointing. Generally speaking, the legislation of mental health law is an essential symbol of a country's civilization and the protection of human rights for the disadvantaged. For this reason, on the basis of understanding the history and development of the protection of the rights of patients with mental disorders in the US, the author boldly proposes some constructive amendments to the Draft.

---

1   This paper is based on the Provisions of the Mental Health Law (Draft) and the Explanations of the Draft published by the website of the National People's Congress of the People's Republic of China on October 29, 2011 as the target material of the study, available at http://www. npc. gov. cn/npc/xinwen/lfgz/flca/ 2011-10/29/content__1678355. htm.

1. Adding a special chapter dedicated to the implementation of "the protection of the rights of patients with mental disorders" to the Draft

The rights of patients with mental disorders should be protected in a legal form. Some of these rights (e.g., the right to privacy) are not unique to mental health service users but are shared by all health service users. However, patients with mental disorders may need special and additional protection because of a long history of being subjected to violations of human rights, stigmatization, and discrimination, and sometimes because of the specific nature of the mental disorder. Patients with mental disorders are sometimes viewed not as adults, but as children, or even as animals. Patients with mental disorders are often considered to lack decision-making capacity, and therefore, their feelings and human dignity are entirely disregarded. The Draft currently contains seven chapters,[1] but no chapter is dedicated to protecting the rights of patients with mental disorders. Many foreign mental health laws (e.g., Brazil, Lithuania, Portugal, Russia, or South Africa) have chapters devoted to the rights of patients with mental disorders, especially the rights of patients with mental disorders in receiving mental health services. In this way, they clarify the specific rights of patients with mental disorders and the legal responsibilities in case of infringements on their rights.[2]

2. Establishing a system to inform patients with mental disorders of their rights in the Draft

In mental health institutions, the rights of patients with mental disorders are more likely to be neglected and violated. Therefore, those who prepare the Draft should learn from the experience of the United States and set up a system of informing patients with mental disorders of their rights in the

---

1   The Draft has seven chapters: General Provisions, Mental Disorder Prevention, Diagnosis and Treatment of Mental Disorders, Rehabilitation of Mental Disorders, Safeguards, Legal Liability, and Supplementary Provisions.

2   *Resource Book on Mental Health, Human Rights and Legislation* (World Health Organization, 2005), 47–53.

Draft. That is to say, any mental health institution shall inform any patient with mental disorders of the rights provided for in the legislation in force when the patient is admitted to or remains in the hospital for observation. Even though the legislation clearly stipulates a number of rights for patients with mental disorders, they are often unaware of the existence of these rights or are not informed about the content of the national legislation. As a result, these patients are incapable of exercising these rights. Therefore, it is necessary to stipulate in the Draft that when a patient receives mental health services, the mental health organization has a statutory obligation to inform the patient of his or her rights in a comprehensive, objective, and effective manner. The mental health organization is required to inform the patient as soon as possible, in a manner and language that the patient fully comprehends, of all his or her rights in accordance with the law. The information should also include an explanation of the rights, how they can be exercised, and specific ways and means of contacting them for protests and complaints. The Draft may even stipulate that the obligation of statutory notification be fulfilled by developing uniformly designed brochures for notification of rights, posters, and videos throughout the country. The Connecticut Department of Mental Health & Addiction Services has issued a Statement of Your Rights as a Client or Patient, and the State of Maine has issued a Statement of Rights of Patients with Mental Disorders. If the patient is incapable of understanding this information, the mental health institution shall inform the patient's representative of the patient's rights. If necessary, the mental health institution may also notify anyone who can best represent the patient's interests and is willing to do so.

3. Refining the protection of patients with mental disorders' rights to communication and visitation in the Draft

In practice, many mental health facilities restrict private meetings between patients and their family members (including their spouses and friends). Their correspondence is often subject to surveillance, with letters being unsealed and, in some cases, scrutinized. Article 42 of the Draft explicitly stipulates the rights of patients with mental disorders to communication and visitation. That is, medical institutions and their medical staff should respect the rights of patients with mental disorders to communicate and meet with visitors, and they should truthfully inform patients or their guardians about the treatment of their illnesses. Based on the current provisions, implementation details should be added to the Draft, such as additional provisions on freedom of communication. These should include the freedom to communicate with others in the mental health facility and the freedom to send and receive personal communications that are not subject to censorship. Furthermore, patients should have the right to request a separate place for meetings when meeting with lawyers and representatives, as well as the freedom to receive other visitors at any reasonable time. They should also have the right to postal, telephone, and Internet services, as well as the right to read newspapers, listen to the radio, and watch television.

Article 42 of the Draft restricts the rights of patients with mental disorders to communication and visitation, i.e., except for the restriction of the rights of patients with mental disorders to communicate and to meet with visitors for the implementation of therapeutic measures. The US legislation is more detailed and specific than the Draft. In order to prevent such restrictive provisions from being abused by mental health facilities in the course of their implementation, it is suggested that the Draft stipulates that the patient's right to communication may be restricted only if there are sufficient grounds to justify that unrestricted communication may jeopardize the patient's health or future prospects, or that such communication may infringe on the rights and freedoms of others. For example, a patient may make repeated unpleasant phone calls or send letters to others, or a depressed person may write or intend to write a letter of resignation to his or her boss. The Draft should also specify additional avenues of relief for patients with mental disorders to appeal these restrictions.

4. Improving the protection of the right to informed consent for patients with mental disorders in the Draft

Articles 35 and 39 of the Draft provide for the right of informed consent for patients with mental disorders. However, it is suggested to refer to the 1972 legislation of the United States to refine the details of the right of informed consent of patients with mental disorders. It should include patients' right to be informed of their own diagnosis, the nature and risks of treatment, the prognosis of not receiving treatment, and the treatment alternatives.

The Draft should be supplemented with the provision that patients with mental disorders shall be entitled to have access to clinical records kept in mental health facilities and by psychiatric professionals. This right should also be limited to prevent serious harm to the patient's health and to avoid threats to the safety of others. The mental health facility should disclose to the patient's representative or attorney any information that cannot be made available to the patient without violating the right to privacy and confidentiality. If any information is withheld from the patient, the mental health facility should inform the patient or the patient's attorney of the reasons for the withholding. An explanation written by the patient or the patient's representative or attorney should be placed in the patient's medical record for future reference.

There are special circumstances in which disclosure of a patient's clinical records could pose a threat to the safety of others or seriously jeopardize the patient's mental health. For example, clinical records may contain information about a patient with a severe disorder from a third party, such as a relative or another physician. Such information, if disclosed to the patient at a particular moment, could cause a severe relapse or even cause the patient to harm themselves or others. Therefore, the Draft should be supplemented by a provision granting professionals the right to withhold such records. The withholding of such information can only be done on a temporary basis, until the moment when the patient is capable of dealing with the information in a reasonable manner.

5. Supplementing the provisions on protecting the rights of patients with mental disorders to work and to be paid for their work in the Draft

The United States has devoted considerable attention in its legislation to the prohibition of employment discrimination against patients with mental disorders. Even today, some states in the US have legislation that explicitly supports some patients with mental disorders being able to work as internists. Moreover, in the current treatment of patients with mental disorders, the concept of "returning to the community" is also advocated, suggesting that patients with mental disorders should be helped to return to society as soon as possible. However, there are not enough provisions in the Draft to protect the labor rights of patients with mental disorders, and only fundamental provisions are made in Article 4.[1]

Given the current situation in China, it is common for people to have misconceptions and discriminatory attitudes towards patients with mental disorders. As a result, it is a prominent problem that patients with mental disorders are discriminated against in employment. It is recommended that the Draft should establish a mechanism for examining whether an employer has discriminated against patients with mental disorders in employment. In particular, it should be specified that the current labor arbitration agencies and people's courts commission judicial appraisal agencies to conduct appraisals on such issues, assessing the employability of patients with mental disorders and whether they are competent to perform their current jobs. At the same time, the Draft should stipulate that injuries to other people's persons and property caused by patients with mental disorders during their work should be included in the scope of compensation by work-related injury insurance. Drawing on the experience of the United States, work-related injury insurance agencies should be allowed to set up a relief fund for accidental injuries of patients with mental disorders to raise charitable funds from the community. Only by eliminating the worries of employers can we fundamentally reduce the employment discrimination against patients with mental disorders.

Article 37 of the Draft stipulates that medical institutions may not force patients with mental disorders to engage in productive labor for purposes other than treatment. In practice, this provision is easily misunderstood as a way of forcing patients with mental disorders to engage in productive work if it is for therapeutic purposes. It is clearly contrary to the principle of eliminating forced labor, a fundamental principle of mental health legislation in the international arena. Forced labor should not be confused with occupational therapy, nor with rehabilitation programs in which patients are asked to make their own beds or prepare food for their peers. However, it is an

---

1 Article 4: "The human dignity and personal safety of patients with mental disorders shall be inviolable, and the lawful rights and interests of patients with mental disorders in education, labor, medical care, protection of privacy, and acquisition of material assistance from the State and society shall be protected by law."

internationally agreed principle that patients with mental disorders should not be forced to work in any circumstance.[1] Patients with mental disorders should have the option of choosing the job type they wish to engage in, even if the needs of the patient are consistent with the management requirements of the mental health facility. Therefore, the Draft should add that mental health institutions should establish facilities and encourage using them to enable patients to actively engage in work that is compatible with their social and cultural background. Furthermore, appropriate vocational rehabilitation and training measures should be adopted to facilitate the reintegration of patients into society. These measures should include vocational guidance, vocational training, and placement services.

The Draft should be supplemented by the provision that patients with mental disorders shall be entitled to be paid for their work, and that the work of patients with mental disorders in mental health institutions may not be exploited. Each patient is entitled to be paid for his or her work and receive the same amount as would be paid by law to a sane person for performing that job.

6. Adding the provisions on the least restrictive protection of the rights of patients with mental disorders for chemical medication to the Draft

Article 36 of the Draft stipulates that medical institutions and their medical staff may impose protective medical measures, such as restraint or seclusion, if patients with mental disorders have committed or are about to commit an act of harming themselves, endangering the safety of others, or disrupting the order of medical treatment within the medical institution, and if restraint or seclusion is the only available means. It can be seen that in terms of physical restraint or seclusion, the Draft follows the principle of the least restriction for patients with mental disorders. However, the Draft does not follow this principle in the use of chemical drugs. Instead, it is only stipulated in Article 37 that the use of drugs for patients with mental disorders

---

1   *Resource Book on Mental Health, Human Rights and Legislation* (World Health Organization, 2005), 47–53.

should be aimed at diagnosis and treatment, safe and effective drugs should be used, and drugs should not be used for purposes other than diagnosis or treatment. It obviously broadens the scope of mandatory drug use. In reality, the use of chemical drugs not only produces the same results as physical restraints or seclusion, but may also cause adverse drug reactions in patients with mental disorders. Therefore, the scope of application of chemical drugs should be as stringent as that of physical restraints or seclusion. The Draft should be supplemented with provisions restricting the use of electro-convulsive therapy, as such therapies are extremely painful and are administered by coercive means. In conclusion, the compulsory use of chemical drugs and electro-convulsive therapy should be restricted to the circumstances specified in Article 36 of the Draft.

7. Strengthening the protection of the rights of patients with mental disorders to refuse medical treatment in the Draft

The doctrine of involuntary commitment and treatment (IC&T) is a long-established theory in the medical community, but it is fraught with problems. Historically, IC&T has been abused and widely criticized for its use against political dissidents in the former Soviet Union.[1] There are also lengthy and sometimes life-long prison sentences for people with mental illness in many Western countries.[2] For this reason, mental health legislation in all countries provides explicit guidelines for the use of IC&T for patients with mental disorders, and procedures are in place to protect IC&T from abuse. The use of IC&T for patients with mental disorders in China has long been a point of contention between psychiatrists and legal workers.[3]

Article 25 of the Draft specifies that the principle of voluntary commitment shall be applied to the hospitalization of patients with mental disorders in China. If the diagnostic conclusion or assessment of the patient's

---

1   K. Fulford et al., "Concepts of Disease and the Abuse of Psychiatry in the USSR," *The British Journal of Psychiatry*, no. 162 (1993): 801–810.

2   G. Grob, "Abuse in American Mental Hospitals in Historical Perspective: Myth and Reality," *International Journal of Law and Psychiatry*, no. 3 (1980): 295–310.

3   L. Burti, "Italian Psychiatric Reform 20 Plus Years After," *Acta Psychiatrica Scandinavica Supplementum*, no. 410 (2001): 41–46.

condition indicates that the patient suffers from severe mental disorders and falls into one of the following categories, the patient should be committed to inpatient treatment: the patient has already committed an act that harms him/herself or is at risk of harming himself/herself, or it is not conducive to the treatment of the patient if he/she is not institutionalized; the patient has already committed an act that jeopardizes the safety of other people or is at risk of jeopardizing the safety of others. For involuntary treatment, the dangerousness principle is adopted in the Draft. However, from the mainstream viewpoint of the current American practice, it is clear that "the dangerousness principle" is unnecessary and unethical, and the adoption of "the dangerousness principle" might cause potential harm to patients with mental diseases and other people. Would we accept the deprivation of liberty of persons suspected of, or likely to commit, crimes that would jeopardize the safety of others? If we have to adopt the dangerousness principle as a criterion for deciding to keep patients with mental diseases under observation, we have to recognize that it may be possible to classify patients with mental disorders throughout the country as requiring compulsory intervention in order to prevent them from causing serious harm. It is undoubtedly discriminatory against patients with mental disorders.

8. Adding provisions on the right to freedom of religious belief of patients with mental disorders to the Draft

At present, the Draft does not contain a specific provision to protect the right to freedom of religious belief of patients with mental disorders. In reality, the protection of this right is of great practical significance. For example, in the case of Zou Yijun in Shenzhen, the right of a patient suspected of having mental disorders was forcibly institutionalized for observation, and her right to Buddhist beliefs was not guaranteed, or even her basic requirement of a vegetarian diet was not fulfilled. It directly led the patient suspected of having mental disorders to go on a hunger strike during the observation period. In fact, it would rather affect the clinician's observation and judgment of the patient's demeanor. For this reason, it is recommended that the Draft should be supplemented with a provision on the right of patients with mental disorders to freedom of religious belief.

9. Supplementing the Draft with the provisions on the right of patients with mental disorders to participate in elections

Currently, the Draft has no provision on whether patients with mental disorders have the right to participate in elections. At present, it is generally believed among the public that patients with mental disorders are not capable of taking part in or being competent in electoral affairs. However, except for patients with mental disorders who do not have cognitive capacity, the majority of patients with mental disorders have full capacity. In view of the fact that China is now rapidly advancing the reform of its democratic electoral system, it is of great practical significance to make specific provisions in the Draft. In the Draft, patients with mental disorders should also be allowed to participate in elections in absentia.

10. Paying more attention to the protection of the right to privacy of patients with mental disorders in the Draft

Privacy in this context has a broader meaning, depending on the extent to which society is involved in individual affairs. It should cover informational, physical, communication, and territorial privacy. These rights of patients with mental disorders may frequently be violated, especially in mental health facilities. For example, patients may be forced to spend many years in dormitory-like wards where they have little space for privacy. They may have no facilities, such as cupboards, to store their personal belongings. Even if a patient is assigned a single or double room, the staff or other patients may feel free to invade the patient's personal space. Privacy and confidentiality should be one of the principles of the legislation of the Draft, meaning that the right to confidentiality of information of all persons covered by the legislation should be respected. At the same time, the Draft should mandate respect for patients' physical privacy and require mental health facilities to be built to make such respect possible. Although China is a developing country with limited resources, it is essential to add to the Draft that the facilities and premises of mental health institutions should be equipped in such a way that privacy protection is not inferior to that of other healthcare institutions.

Articles 4, 18, 42, and 70 of the Draft address the issue of privacy protection for patients with mental disorders. However, there are apparent problems with the exceptions to the right to privacy. The exceptions to the right to privacy cover the circumstances under which information about a person with a mental disorder may be disclosed to another party without the prior consent of the person. It is of great practical significance. Although the Draft provides for this in Article 42,[1] it is clearly too narrow by only including the performance of duties by the executive branch in accordance with the law as an exception to the protection of the right to privacy. It is recommended to follow the example of the US legislation. On the one hand, it should be made clear that child abuse and the mental state of patients with mental disorders as part of administrative law enforcement or judicial proceedings should fall within the scope of the exception to privacy protection. On the other hand, it should be made clear that the content of communications between physicians and patients, even if they include attempts to commit a crime or harmful acts, should fall within the scope of privacy protection and should not be disclosed unless the statutory conditions of the first dimension are met. In addition, it is proposed that the Draft should specify that administrators of mental health facilities should ensure that appropriate procedures and systems are in place to protect patients' privacy. It implies that an effective system needs to be put in place to guarantee that only authorized persons have access to a patient's clinical records or other data records, such as electronic medical record databases.

The Draft must consider "deinstitutionalization" as an essential initiative and system for protecting the privacy of patients with mental disorders. If appropriate services are provided in the community, deinstitutionalization can be a valid way of freeing many patients from the crowded and impersonal hospital environment and providing them with a greater level of privacy.

The right to privacy in mental health facilities does not mean that patients cannot be subjected to protective searches or continued close observation in special circumstances, such as when they attempt to commit suicide. Limitations on the right to privacy in these circumstances should be

---

1   Article 42: "Without the consent of the patient or his/her guardian, no unit or individual may disclose the name, address, workplace, portrait, medical records, or any other information that might reveal the identity of the patient or his/her family members; however, there are exceptions for those that are required to be disclosed by the administrative authorities in the performance of their duties in accordance with the law."

carefully considered against the internationally recognized standards of the right. For this reason, it is proposed that the Draft should be supplemented with exceptions to privacy disclosures that may be lawful. These include situations where the information is urgently needed to save a life in a life-threatening emergency, where there is a substantial likelihood of serious harm or injury to the patient or others, where it is necessary to prevent an apparent epidemic, and where it is required to protect the interests of public safety.

11. Refining the provisions on protecting the right of patients with mental disorders to receive periodic review in the Draft

Articles 40, 45, and 48 of the Draft establish a mechanism for periodic supervision and review of patients with mental disorders. The main bodies of these mechanisms are differentiated, being medical institutions, county-level health administrative departments and community health service organizations, township (town) health centers, and village health rooms, respectively. However, based on past cases of long-term incarceration of patients with mental disorders in China, these three types of institutions have a complex relationship of interest and achievements with local governments. Furthermore, their neutrality and impartiality are questionable. For this reason, the Draft should be supplemented with a provision that public welfare organizations or any individuals shall be allowed to participate in the above-mentioned appraisal, supervision, and review and shall be entitled to initiate the investigation and assessment of whether patients with mental disorders need to continue to be institutionalized or not.

Mental health is both a major global public health issue and a prominent social one. For a long time, the vast number of patients with mental disorders in China have suffered from the pain of illness, prejudice, and discrimination. As one of the most vulnerable groups in society, they are not fully protected in terms of their legal rights and interests and human dignity, and they are in a low social status and very miserable conditions. It is hoped that the Mental Health Law of the People's Republic of China will be enacted as soon as possible to effectively protect the rights of patients with mental disorders.

A Comparative Study of the Mental Health Law of the People's Republic of China and WHO Legislative Proposals

I. Introduction

Mental health is not only a major public health issue around the globe, but also a prominent social issue. Mental health legislation in China has been a topic of health legislation followed closely by society and scholars. To start with, the issue of mental health is especially prominent in China. Mental illnesses rank first in the total burden of diseases in China, accounting for 20% thereof. According to WHO sampling analysis of people aged 15–44 in the world, social burdens caused by mental disorders account for 1/4 of the total social burden of diseases, and 5 of the 10 diseases causing maximum functional defects are mental disorders. A survey by the Ministry of Health shows that over 100 million people in China now suffer from mental disorders, including about 16 million suffering from severe mental illnesses.[1] Due to unknown etiology and pathogenesis, most mental disorders cannot be prevented or treated in a targeted way, leading to a low cure rate of mental disorders and a high rate of disability. Because of mental disorders, some patients may even have unpredictable behaviors such as committing suicide,

---

1   "CINP Asia-Pacific Regional Meeting Pointed Out New Drugs for Common Mental Disorders Greatly Improved the Prognosis," *China Medical Tribune*, April 8, 2004.

injuring themselves or other people, or destroying property, which not only cause heavy burdens to themselves and their families, but also potentially harm society. Secondly, the numerous patients suffering from mental disorders in China have been tortured by illnesses, prejudice, and discrimination for a long. Though people suffering from mental disorders are one of the most disadvantaged social groups, their legitimate rights and interests and dignity of human personality cannot be fully protected, their social status is low, and their conditions are miserable. Besides, mental disorders are an important reason that some urban and rural households become impoverished again. Thirdly, mental health management is different from other forms of medical services. Mental disorders are special not only in prevention, diagnosis, and treatment, but also in rehabilitation and management, since patients of mental illnesses normally seek treatment with the assistance of their guardians or forced by the public security organ; besides some very special ways of treatment, many drugs for treating mental illnesses lead to adverse reactions that are intolerable for ordinary people. During the attack of mental illnesses, patients normally lose the ability to express themselves. They cannot make rational and reasonable decisions or control their behaviors, so they have to be placed under physical restraints or seclusion, confined in handling their personal affairs, or given mandatory treatment, etc. Mental illness patients, under the control of psychotic symptoms, often have unexpected dangerous behaviors or are exposed to accidents of all kinds for which mental health workers always feel powerless, and even place their lives and property at great risk. The above features put mental health work in front of high risks, and a great number of legal issues and disputes, the legislation of which has been blank and needs to be adjusted via special legislation.

In 1985, the Ministry of Health of China appointed the Sichuan Provincial Department of Health to take the lead and the Hunan Provincial Department of Health to assist in drawing up Mental Health Law (Draft) together. However, due to great controversies over some legal issues, it was not deliberated, passed, and promulgated by the National People's Congress. In this period, Shanghai formulated the first mental health-related local statute—Shanghai Mental Health Regulations. As of April 2010, eight places in China had developed local regulations on mental health. Shanghai, Ningbo, Beijing, Hangzhou, and Wuxi developed mental health regulations in succession; Shanghai, Dalian, Heilongjiang, and Shijiazhuang developed local regulations on intensive care, treatment, and management of mental patients causing trouble or accidents.

From 1998 to 2008, the media reported 24 cases involving the protection of rights for people suffering from mental illnesses (these include the case of Liu Yalin killing children, the case of Chen Jian'an killing his brothers, the case of Zhu Jinhong in Jiangsu, the case of He Jinrong in Guangzhou, the case of Zou Yijun in Shenzhen, etc.). Amidst powerful social opinions, the Chinese legislature continued to advance the work of drawing up the Mental Health Law. Eventually, after over 20 revisions in 26 years, Mental Health Law (Draft) was officially released on June 10, 2011, and public opinions were solicited. It was passed at the 29th meeting of the Standing Committee of the Eleventh National People's Congress on October 26, 2012, and formally implemented on May 1, 2013.

It should be said that the promulgation of the Mental Health Law is an event of milestone significance to the mental health cause in China. It will undoubtedly correct and intervene in the chaotic situation of a lack of central legislation for a long time. Yet, it is criticized by different social sectors, for people think that many contents are not detailed and operable. The paper takes the WHO Checklist on Mental Health Legislation in the *Resource Book on Mental Health, Human Rights and Legislation* (WHO, 2005) as the study tool. It means discovering the deficiencies of the Mental Health Law of the People's Republic of China in the aspect of protecting human rights in the hope of further improving it in later legislation.

According to Muir Gray, the task of the medical industry is not only maintaining and improving industrial achievements of modern times, but also making due adjustments along with social development. Its focus should be shifted from "phenomenon evidence" to "value system," and its point of interest should be shifted from "interests" to "challenging itself." As a matter of fact, the medical industry has completed the change and begun to accept it. However, in the domain of mental health, there is another difficulty that will never be faced by other medical specialties, and the achievements made by it in the 20th century are also doubted. For example, people have been complaining about waiting too long in a hospital, being badly treated by medical service staff, and communicating inefficiently with doctors, but few doubt medical technologies themselves. Psychiatry in the 20th century had been challenged and doubted by the public.[1] We cannot imagine that the public would launch the "anti-pediatric" movement or the movement to "criticize anesthesiology." However, the "anti-psychiatry" movement and the movement to "criticize psychiatry" have a long history. Psychiatry in the 20th century had been conservatively resisting such challenges and building its own medical characteristics. Though the subject survived the resistance movement in the 1960s, there are root legal and moral issues to be solved. Against such background, this paper, by taking the degree of consistency between the WHO Checklist on Mental Health Legislation and Mental Health Law as the point of entry, tries to further explore the current major problems of Mental Health Law and propose improvement suggestions.

II. Research Methods

A comparison is made on the provisions of China's first Mental Health Law (2012) following the national mental health legislation requirements in the *Resource Book on Mental Health, Human Rights and Legislation* (WHO, 2005). Since Mental Health Law was officially implemented on May 1, 2013, there is insufficient evidence to evaluate the effect of its implementation thoroughly. Hence, this study only makes a comparative analysis of the legislative contents instead of the legislative implementation effect.

In the annexes to *Resource Book on Mental Health, Human Rights and Legislation,* there is a detailed WHO Checklist on Mental Health Legislation, which is for the reference of different countries in legislation and aims at institutionalizing the protection of human rights to the maximum extent. The list includes 166 components and 27 categories (A–AZ) (see the table below). WHO Checklist on Mental Health Legislation also provides a useful tool for legislation and review, and thus is conducive to promoting different countries' national mental health legislation.

For each component included in the checklist, the extent to which it is covered by legislation needs to be addressed: a) adequately covered, b) covered to some extent, and c) not covered at all. If the response is either (b) or

---

1   T. Szasz, *The Myth of Mental Illness* (New York: Harper and Row, 1961).

(c), this paper will analyze major issues later in the hope of advancing and improving mental health legislation in China in the future.

III. Major Problems Discovered in the Comparison and Suggestions

As seen from the history of mental health legislation in different countries, mental health legislation is the most controversial work in health legislation, so progressive mental health legislation prevails in different countries. Many countries in America and Europe, led by the UK, have also begun to change the nature of the mental health sector by constantly adjusting their national policies and legislation. To address the relations between poverty, unemployment, and mental disorders, national policies and legislation have begun to pay attention to disadvantaged groups and the issue of social exclusion.[1] Within the "national mental health service policy and legal framework," different countries have begun to highlight the importance of the social environment, the value system, and collaboration. The change is undoubtedly a reflection of and challenge against modern psychiatry under the traditional biomedical model.[2] In short, different countries' governments and peoples are all eager to reform the relationship between psychiatry and its practitioners and the service objects.[3] WHO Checklist on Mental Health Legislation undoubtedly provides a platform of communication for different countries to constantly improve their mental health legislation and a tool for them to amend laws. According to the above comparative analysis, the Chinese Mental Health Law conforms to 62 components of the 166 components of the WHO Checklist on Mental Health Legislation on the protection of human rights (the rate of consistency is 37.3%). Some foreign scholars also adopted the same research method to compare the legislation in their coun-

---

1   Department of Health, *Saving Lives: Our Healthier Nation* (London: Stationery Office, 1998).

2   Ibid., *Modern Standards and Service Models: Mental Health* (London: Stationery Office, 1999).

3   Muir Gray J. A., "Postmodern Medicine," *Lancet*, no. 354 (1999): 1550–1553.

tries with WHO standards on the protection of human rights. The studies of Kelly show that mental health legislation in England & Wales conforms to 90 components of the 166 components of the WHO Checklist on Mental Health Legislation (the rate of consistency is 48.2%), while that in Ireland conforms to 80 components (the rate of consistency is 48.2%).[1] As can be seen, there is much room for perfecting some terms in Mental Health Law in China.

Table 2. WHO checklist on mental health legislation

Legislative issue	Extent to which covered in legislation (tick one) a) Adequately covered b) Covered to some extent c) Not covered at all			Mental Health Law of the People's Republic of China
A. Preamble and objectives				
1) Does the legislation have a preamble which emphasizes:				
a) the human rights of people with mental disorders?	a)	b)	c)	A1, A4.
b) the importance of accessible mental health services for all?	a)	b)	c)	A2
2) Does the legislation specify that the purpose and objectives to be achieved include:				
a) non-discrimination against people with mental disorders?	a)	b)	c)	A5
b) promotion and protection of the rights of people with mental disorders?	a)	b)	c)	A1, A4–5.
c) improved access to mental health services?	a)	b)	c)	A2–4, A26.
d) a community-based approach?	a)	b)	c)	A20, A54–55, A61, A63

---

1   Brendan D. Kelly, "Mental Health Legislation and Human Rights in England, Wales, and the Republic of Ireland," *International Journal of Law and Psychiatry* 34, no. 6 (November–December 2011): 439–454.

B. Definitions

	a)	b)	c)	
1) Is there a clear definition of mental disorder/mental illness/mental disability/mental incapacity?	a)	**b)**	c)	A83
2) Is it evident from the legislation why the particular term (above) has been chosen?	a)	b)	c)	
3) Is the legislation clear on whether or not mental retardation/intellectual disability, personality disorders, and substance abuse are being covered in the legislation?	a)	b)	c)	
4) Are all key terms in the legislation clearly defined?	a)	b)	c)	
5) Are all the key terms used consistently throughout the legislation (i.e., not interchanged with other terms with similar meanings)?	a)	b)	c)	
6) Are all "interpretable" terms (i.e., terms that may have several possible interpretations or meanings or may be ambiguous in terms of their meaning) in the legislation defined?	a)	b)	c)	

C. Access to mental healthcare

	a)	b)	c)	
1) Does the legislation make provision for the financing of mental health services?	a)	b)	c)	A62–63
2) Does the legislation state that mental health services should be provided on an equal basis with physical healthcare?	a)	b)	c)	
3) Does the legislation ensure the allocation of resources to underserved populations and specify that these services should be culturally appropriate?	a)	b)	c)	A69
4) Does the legislation promote mental health within primary healthcare?	a)	b)	c)	A63
5) Does the legislation promote access to psychotropic drugs?	a)	b)	c)	A41
6) Does the legislation promote a psychosocial, rehabilitative approach?	a)	b)	c)	A13
7) Does the legislation promote access to health insurance in the private and public health sectors for people with mental disorders?	a)	b)	c)	

8) Does the legislation promote community care and deinstitutionalization?	a)	b)	c)	A20, A54–55, A61, A63
D. Rights of users of mental health services				
1) Does the legislation include the rights to respect, dignity and to be treated in a humane way?	a)	b)	c)	A5, A26
2) Is the right to patients' confidentiality regarding information about themselves, their illness, and treatment included?				
a) Are there sanctions and penalties for people who contravene patients' confidentiality?	a)	b)	c)	A78
b) Does the legislation lay down exceptional circumstances when confidentiality may be legally breached?	a)	b)	c)	A27
c) Does the legislation allow patients and their personal representatives the right to ask for judicial review of, or appeal against, decisions to release information?	a)	b)	c)	A82
3) Does the legislation provide patients free and full access to information about themselves (including access to their clinical records)?				
a) Are circumstances in which such access can be denied outlined?	a)	b)	c)	A47
b) Does the legislation allow patients and their personal representatives the right to ask for judicial review of, or appeal against, decisions to withhold information?	a)	b)	c)	A82
4) Does the law specify the right to be protected from cruel, inhuman, and degrading treatment?	a)	b)	c)	A9, A40–43
5) Does the legislation set out the minimal conditions to be maintained in mental health facilities for a safe, therapeutic and hygienic environment?	a)	b)	c)	A38
6) Does the law insist on the privacy of people with mental disorders?				

	a)	b)	c)	
a) Is the law clear on minimal levels of privacy to be respected?	a)	**b)**	c)	A27
7) Does the legislation outlaw forced or inadequately remunerated labour within mental health institutions?	**a)**	b)	c)	A41
8) Does the law make provision for: • educational activities, • vocational training, • leisure and recreational activities, and • religious or cultural needs of people with mental disorders?	a)	**b)**	c)	A4, A70, A58
9) Are the health authorities compelled by the law to inform patients of their rights?	a)	**b)**	c)	A37
10) Does legislation ensure that users of mental health services are involved in mental health policy, legislation development, and service planning?	a)	b)	**c)**	
E. Rights of families or other carers				
1) Does the law entitle families or other primary carers to information about the person with a mental disorder (unless the patient refuses the divulging of such information)?	**a)**	b)	c)	A39–40, A43–44, A47
2) Are family members or other primary carers encouraged to become involved in the formulation and implementation of the patient's individualized treatment plan?	a)	**b)**	c)	A39–44
3) Do families or other primary carers have the right to appeal involuntary admission and treatment decisions?	**a)**	b)	c)	A28
4) Do families or other primary carers have the right to apply for the discharge of mentally ill offenders?	a)	b)	**c)**	
5) Does legislation ensure that family members or other carers are involved in the development of mental health policy, legislation, and service planning?	a)	b)	**c)**	

F. Competence, capacity, and guardianship

1) Does legislation make provision for the management of the affairs of people with mental disorders if they are unable to do so? — a) b) **c)**

2) Does the law define "competence" and "capacity"? — a) b) c)

3) Does the law lay down a procedure and criteria for determining a person's incapacity/incompetence with respect to issues such as treatment decisions, selection of a substitute decision-maker, and financial decisions? — a) b) c)

4) Are procedures laid down for appeals against decisions of incapacity/ incompetence, and for periodic reviews of decisions? — a) b) **c)**

5) Does the law lay down procedures for the appointment, duration, duties, and responsibilities of a guardian to act on behalf of a patient? — a) b) c)

6) Does the law determine a process for establishing in which areas a guardian may make decisions on behalf of a patient? — a) b) c)

7) Does the law make provision for a systematic review of the need for a guardian? — a) b) **c)**

8) Does the law make provision for a patient to appeal against the appointment of a guardian? — a) b) **c)**

G. Voluntary admission and treatment

1) Does the law promote voluntary admission and treatment as a preferred alternative to involuntary admission and treatment? — **a)** b) c) A30

2) Does the law state that all voluntary patients can only be treated after obtaining informed consent? — a) b) **c)**

3) Does the law state that people admitted as voluntary mental health users should be

cared for in a way that is equitable with patients with physical health problems?	a)	b)	<u>c)</u>	
4) Does the law state that voluntary admission and treatment also imply the right to voluntary discharge/refusal of treatment?	<u>a)</u>	b)	c)	A44
5) Does the law state that voluntary patients should be informed at the time of admission that they may only be denied the right to leave if they meet the conditions for involuntary care?	a)	b)	<u>c)</u>	
H. Non-protesting patients				
1) Does the law make provision for patients who are incapable of making informed decisions about admission or treatment, but who do not refuse admission or treatment?	<u>a)</u>	b)	c)	A28
2) Are the conditions under which a non-protesting patient may be admitted and treated specified?	<u>a)</u>	b)	c)	A28
3) Does the law state that if users admitted or treated under this provision object to their admission or treatment they must be discharged or treatment stopped unless the criteria for involuntary admission are met?	a)	b)	<u>c)</u>	
I. Involuntary admission (when separate from treatment) and involuntary treatment (where admission and treatment are combined)				
1) Does the law state that involuntary admission may only be allowed if:				
a) there is evidence of mental disorder of specified severity? and;	<u>a)</u>	b)	c)	A30
b) there is serious likelihood of harm to self or others and/or substantial likelihood of serious deterioration in the patient's condition if treatment is not given? and;	a)	<u>b)</u>	c)	A30

	a)	b)	c)	
c) admission is for a therapeutic purpose?	a)	b)	<u>c)</u>	
2) Does the law state that two accredited mental healthcare practitioners must certify that the criteria for involuntary admission have been met?	a)	b)	<u>c)</u>	
3) Does the law insist on accreditation of a facility before it can admit involuntary patients?	<u>a)</u>	b)	c)	A29
4) Is the principle of the least restrictive environment applied to involuntary admissions?	a)	b)	<u>c)</u>	
5) Does the law make provision for an independent authority (e.g., review body or tribunal) to authorize all involuntary admissions?	a)	b)	<u>c)</u>	A32
6) Are speedy time frames laid down within which the independent authority must make a decision?	a)	<u>b)</u>	c)	
7) Does the law insist that patients, families, and legal representatives be informed of the reasons for admission and of their rights of appeal?	<u>a)</u>	b)	c)	A37
8) Does the law provide for a right to appeal an involuntary admission?	<u>a)</u>	b)	c)	A32
9) Does the law include a provision for time-bound periodic reviews of involuntary (and long-term "voluntary") admission by an independent authority?	a)	<u>b)</u>	c)	A50
10) Does the law specify that patients must be discharged from involuntary admission as soon as they no longer fulfill the criteria for involuntary admission?	<u>a)</u>	b)	c)	A44
J. Involuntary treatment (when separate from involuntary admission)				
1) Does the law set out the criteria that must be met for involuntary treatment, including:				
• Patient suffers from a mental disorder?	a)	b)	<u>c)</u>	
• Patient lacks the capacity to make informed treatment decisions?	a)	b)	<u>c)</u>	

• Treatment is necessary to bring about an improvement in the patient's condition, and/or restore the capacity to make treatment decisions, and/or prevent serious deterioration, and/or prevent injury or harm to self or others?	a)	b)	<u>c)</u>	
2) Does the law ensure that a treatment plan is proposed by an accredited practitioner with expertise and knowledge to provide the treatment?	<u>a)</u>	b)	c)	A25
3) Does the law make provision for a second practitioner to agree on the treatment plan?	a)	b)	<u>c)</u>	
4) Has an independent body been set up to authorize involuntary treatment?	<u>a)</u>	b)	c)	A50
5) Does the law ensure that treatment is for a limited time period only?	a)	b)	<u>c)</u>	
6) Does the law provide for a right to appeal involuntary treatment?	<u>a)</u>	b)	c)	A28
7) Are there speedy, time-bound, periodic reviews of involuntary treatment in the legislation?	a)	b)	<u>c)</u>	
K. Proxy consent for treatment				
1) Does the law provide for a person to consent to treatment on a patient's behalf if that patient has been found incapable of consenting?	a)	<u>b)</u>	c)	A39
2) Is the patient given the right to appeal a treatment decision to which a proxy consent has been given?	a)	b)	<u>c)</u>	
3) Does the law provide for the use of "advance directives" and, if so, is the term clearly defined?	a)	b)	<u>c)</u>	
L. Involuntary treatment in community settings				
1) Does the law provide for involuntary treatment in the community as a "less restrictive" alternative to an inpatient mental health facility?	a)	b)	<u>c)</u>	

2) Are all the criteria and safeguards required for involuntary inpatient treatment also included for involuntary community-based treatment?	a)	b)	<u>c)</u>	
M. Emergency situavtions				
1) Are the criteria for emergency admission/treatment limited to situations where there is a high probability of immediate and imminent danger or harm to self and/or others?	<u>a)</u>	b)	c)	A28
2) Is there a clear procedure in the law for admission and treatment in emergency situations?	<u>a)</u>	b)	c)	A29
3) Does the law allow any qualified and accredited medical or mental health practitioner to admit and treat emergency cases?	<u>a)</u>	b)	c)	A29
4) Does the law specify a time limit for emergency admission (usually no longer than 72 hours)?	a)	b)	<u>c)</u>	
5) Does the law specify the need to initiate procedures for involuntary admission and treatment, if needed, as soon as possible after the emergency situation has ended?	a)	b)	<u>c)</u>	
6) Are treatments such as ECT, psychosurgery, and sterilization, as well as participation in clinical or experimental trials outlawed for people held as emergency cases?	a)	<u>b)</u>	c)	A42–43
7) Do patients, family members, and personal representatives have the right to appeal against emergency admission/treatment?	a)	b)	<u>c)</u>	
N. Determinations of mental disorder				
1) Does the legislation:				
a) Define the level of skills required to determine mental disorder?	<u>a)</u>	b)	c)	A29
b) Specify the categories of professionals who may assess a person to determine the existence of a mental disorder?	<u>a)</u>	b)	c)	A29

2) Is the accreditation of practitioners codified in law and does this ensure that accreditation is operated by an independent body?	<u>a)</u>	b)	c)	A29
O. Special treatments 1) Does the law prohibit sterilization as a treatment for mental disorders? a) Does the law specify that the mere fact of having a mental disorder should not be a reason for sterilization or abortion without informed consent?	a)	b)	<u>c)</u>	
2) Does the law require informed consent for major medical and surgical procedures on persons with a mental disorder? a) Does the law allow medical and surgical procedures without informed consent, if waiting for informed consent would put the patient's life at risk?	a)	b)	<u>c)</u>	
b) In cases where the inability to consent is likely to be long-term, does the law allow authorization for medical and surgical procedures from an independent review body or by proxy consent of a guardian?	a)	b)	<u>c)</u>	
3) Are psychosurgery and other irreversible treatments outlawed on involuntary patients? a) Is there an independent body that makes sure there is indeed informed consent for psychosurgery or other irreversible treatments on involuntary patients?	<u>a)</u>	b)	c)	A43
4) Does the law specify the need for informed consent when using ECT?	a)	b)	<u>c)</u>	
5) Does the law prohibit the use of unmodified ECT?	a)	b)	<u>c)</u>	
6) Does the law prohibit the use of ECT in minors?	a)	b)	<u>c)</u>	

P. Seclusion and restraint			
1) Does the law state that seclusion and restraint should only be utilized in exceptional cases to prevent immediate or imminent harm to self or others?	<u>a)</u> b) c)		A40
2) Does the law state that seclusion and restraint should never be used as a means of punishment or for the convenience of staff?	<u>a)</u> b) c)		A40
3) Does the law specify a restricted maximum time period for which seclusion and restraints can be used?	a) b) <u>c)</u>		
4) Does the law ensure that one period of seclusion and restraint is not followed immediately by another?	a) b) <u>c)</u>		
5) Does the law encourage the development of appropriate structural and human resource requirements that minimize the need to use seclusion and restraints in mental health facilities?	a) b) <u>c)</u>		
6) Does the law lay down adequate procedures for the use of seclusion and restraints, including: • who should authorize it, • that the facility should be accredited, • that the reasons and duration of each incident be recorded in a database and made available to a review board, and • that family members/carers and personal representatives be immediately informed when the patient is subject to seclusion and/or restraint?	a) <u>b)</u> c)		A50
Q. Clinical and experimental research			
1) Does the law state that informed consent must be obtained for participation in clinical or experimental research from both voluntary and involuntary patients who have the ability to consent?	<u>a)</u> b) c)		A43
2) Where a person is unable to give informed consent (and where a decision has been made that research can be conducted):			

a) Does the law ensure that proxy consent is obtained from either the legally appointed guardian or family member, or from an independent authority constituted for this purpose?	<u>a)</u>	b)	c)	A43
b) Does the law state that the research cannot be conducted if the same research could be conducted on people capable of consenting, and that the research is necessary to promote the health of the individual and that of the population represented?	<u>a)</u>	b)	c)	A43
R. Oversight and review mechanisms 1) Does the law set up a judicial or quasi-judicial body to review processes related to involuntary admission or treatment and other restrictions of rights? a) Does the above body:				
(i) Assess each involuntary admission/treatment?	<u>a)</u>	b)	c)	A50
(ii) Entertain appeals against involuntary admission and/or involuntary treatment?	a)	b)	<u>c)</u>	
(iii) Review the cases of patients admitted on an involuntary basis (and long-term voluntary patients)?	<u>a)</u>	b)	c)	A50
(iv) Regularly monitor patients receiving treatment against their will?	<u>a)</u>	b)	c)	A50
(v) Authorize or prohibit intrusive and irreversible treatments (such as psychosurgery and ECT)?	<u>a)</u>	b)	c)	A50
b) Does the composition of this body include an experienced legal practitioner and an experienced healthcare practitioner, and a "wise person" reflecting the "community" perspective?	a)	b)	<u>c)</u>	
c) Does the law allow for appeal of this body's decisions to a higher court?	a)	b)	<u>c)</u>	
2) Does the law set up a regulatory and oversight body to protect the rights of				

	a)	b)	c)	
people with mental disorders within and outside mental health facilities?				
a) Does the above body:				
(i) Conduct regular inspections of mental health facilities?	<u>a)</u>	b)	c)	A50
(ii) Provide guidance on minimizing intrusive treatments?	a)	b)	<u>c)</u>	
(iii) Maintain statistics; on, for example, the use of intrusive and irreversible treatments, seclusion and restraints?	a)	b)	<u>c)</u>	
(iv) Maintain registers of accredited facilities and professionals?	<u>a)</u>	b)	c)	A29
(v) Report and make recommendations directly to the appropriate government minister?	a)	b)	<u>c)</u>	
(vi) Publish findings on a regular basis?	a)	b)	<u>c)</u>	
b) Does the composition of the body include professionals (in mental health, legal, and social work), representatives of users of mental health facilities, members representing families of people with mental disorders, advocates, and lay persons?	a)	b)	<u>c)</u>	
c) Is this body's authority clearly stated in the legislation?	<u>a)</u>	b)	c)	A50
3)				
a) Does the legislation outline procedures for submissions, investigations, and resolutions of complaints?	a)	b)	<u>c)</u>	
b) Does the law stipulate:				
• the time period from the occurrence of the incident within which the complaint should be made?	a)	b)	<u>c)</u>	
• a maximum time period within which the complaint should be responded to, by whom and how?	a)	b)	<u>c)</u>	
• the right of patients to choose and appoint a personal representative and/or legal counsel to represent them in any appeals or complaints procedures?	a)	b)	<u>c)</u>	
• the right of patients to an interpreter during the proceedings, if necessary?	a)	b)	<u>c)</u>	

• The right of patients and their counsel to access copies of their medical records and any other relevant reports and documents during the complaints or appeals procedures?	a)	b)	c)	
• the right of patients and their counsel to attend and participate in complaints and appeals procedures?	a)	b)	c)	
S. Police responsibilities				
1) Does the law place restrictions on the activities of the police to ensure that persons with mental disorders are protected against unlawful arrest and detention, and are directed towards the appropriate healthcare services?	a)	b)	c)	
2) Does the legislation allow family members, carers, or health professionals to obtain police assistance in situations where a patient is highly aggressive or is showing out-of-control behaviour?	a)	b)	c)	A28, A35
3) Does the law allow for persons arrested for criminal acts, and in police custody, to be promptly assessed for mental disorder if there is suspicion of mental disorder?	a)	b)	c)	
4) Does the law make provision for the police to assist in taking a person to a mental health facility who has been involuntarily admitted to the facility?	a)	b)	c)	A35
5) Does the legislation make provision for the police to find an involuntarily committed person who has absconded and return him/her to the mental health facility?	a)	b)	c)	A35
T. Mentally ill offenders				
1) Does the legislation allow for diverting an alleged offender with a mental disorder to the mental health system in lieu of prosecuting him/her, taking into account the gravity of the offence, the person's psychiatric history, mental health state at the time of the offence, the likelihood of				

detriment to the person's health and the community's interest in prosecution?	a)	b)	c)	A53
2) Does the law make adequate provision for people who are not fit to stand trial to be assessed, and for charges to be dropped or stayed while they undergo treatment?				
a) Are people undergoing such treatment given the same rights in the law as other involuntarily admitted persons, including the right to judicial review by an independent body?	a)	b)	c)	
3) Does the law allow for people who are found by the courts to be "not responsible due to mental disability" to be treated in a mental health facility and to be discharged once their mental disorder sufficiently improves?	a)	b)	c)	
4) Does the law allow, at the sentencing stage, for persons with mental disorders to be given probation or hospital orders, rather than being sentenced to prison?	a)	b)	c)	
5) Does the law allow for the transfer of a convicted prisoner to a mental health facility if he/she becomes mentally ill while serving a sentence?	a)	b)	c)	
a) Does the law prohibit keeping a prisoner in the mental health facility for longer than the sentence, unless involuntary admission procedures are followed?	a)	b)	c)	
6) Does the legislation provide for secure mental health facilities for mentally ill offenders?	a)	b)	c)	
U. Discrimination				
1) Does the law include provisions aimed at stopping discrimination against people with mental disorders?	a)	b)	c)	A5
V. Housing				
1) Does the law ensure non-discrimination of people with mental disorders in the allocation of housing?	a)	b)	c)	

2) Does the law make provision for housing of people with mental disorders in state housing schemes or through subsidized housing?	a)	b)	c)	
3) Does the legislation make provision for housing in halfway homes and long-stay, supported homes for people with mental disorders?	a)	b)	c)	
W. Employment				
1) Does the law make provision for the protection of persons with mental disorders from discrimination and exploitation in the work place?	a)	b)	c)	A5, A58
2) Does the law provide for "reasonable accommodation" for employees with mental disorders, for example by providing for a degree of flexibility in working hours to enable those employees to seek mental health treatment?	a)	b)	c)	A58
3) Does the law provide for equal employment opportunities for people with mental disorders?	a)	b)	c)	
4) Does the law make provision for the establishment of vocational rehabilitation programmes and other programmes that provide jobs and employment in the community for people with mental discorders?	a)	b)	c)	A58, A70
X. Social security				
1) Does legislation provide for disability grants and pensions for people with mental disabilities?	a)	b)	c)	A69
2) Does the law provide for disability grants and pensions for people with mental disorders at similar rates as those for people with physical disabilities?	a)	b)	c)	
Y. Civil issues				
1) Does the law uphold the rights of people with mental disorders to the full range				

of civil, political, economic, social, and cultural rights to which all people are entitled?	a)	b)	c)	
Z. Protection of vulnerable groups *Protection of minors* 1) Does the law limit the involuntary placement of minors in mental health facilities to instances where all feasible community alternatives have been tried?	a)	b)	c)	
2) If minors are placed in mental health facilities, does the legislation stipulate that a) they should have a separate living area from adults?	a)	b)	c)	
b) that the environment is age-appropriate and takes into consideration the developmental needs of minors?	a)	b)	c)	
3) Does the law ensure that all minors have an adult to represent them in all matters affecting them, including consenting to treatment?	a)	b)	c)	
4) Does the law stipulate the need to take the opinions of minors into consideration on all issues affecting them (including consent to treatment), depending on their age and maturity?	a)	b)	c)	
5) Does legislation ban all irreversible treatments for children?	a)	b)	c)	
Protection of women 1) Does legislation allow women with mental disorders equal rights with men in all matters relating to civil, political, economic, social, and cultural rights?	a)	b)	c)	
2) Does the law ensure that women in mental health facilities: a) have adequate privacy?	a)	b)	c)	
b) are provided with separate sleeping facilities from men?	a)	b)	c)	
3) Does legislation state that women with mental disorders should receive equal mental health treatment and care as				

men, including access to mental health services and care in the community, and in relation to voluntary and involuntary admission and treatment?	a)	b)	c)
Protection of minorities			
1) Does legislation specifically state that persons with mental disorders should not be discriminated against on the grounds of race, colour, language, religion, political or other opinions, national, ethnic or social origin, legal or social status?	a)	b)	c)
2) Does the legislation provide for a review body to monitor involuntary admission and treatment of minorities and ensure non-discrimination on all matters?	a)	b)	c)
3) Does the law stipulate that refugees and asylum seekers are entitled to the same mental health treatment as other citizens of the host country?	a)	b)	c)
AZ. Offences and penalties			
1) Does the law have a section dealing with offences and appropriate penalties?	a)	b)	c)	A81
2) Does the law provide appropriate sanctions against individuals who violate any of the rights of patients as established in the law?	a)	b)	c)	A82

1. Issues in such aspects as definition, legal capacity, and guardianship (B, F)

Mental disorders, mental illnesses, and mental incapacity are very confusing concepts covering different scopes. If the legislation is on involuntary treatment and other restricted rights only, it is better to use the concept with a narrower meaning (mental incapacity). If the legislation also provides anti-discrimination and health promotion content and similar content on the protection of rights and interests, a more inclusive concept (mental disorder) can protect the rights and interests of more extensive groups of people. Another feasible practice is to use a broader concept on the whole, but a narrower concept in the involuntary treatment part. In its Supplementary Articles, Mental Health Law defines both "mental disorder" and "people suffering from severe mental disorders." It makes "severe mental disorders" a precondition for involuntary treatment, yet it fails to define "mental incapacity." Though "capacity" is a concept that already exists in the General Principles of the Civil Law of the People's Republic of China, Mental Health Law avoids it instead of properly linking it with the declaration system of capacity for civil conduct and civil guardian system under the current Civil Law of the People's Republic of China; thus, it is impossible to well solve the phenomenon of "being treated as a psychotic" frequently occurring in the society. In the Supplementary Articles of Mental Health Law, "a mentally disordered person's guardian, as referred to in this law, refers to one who may assume guardianship under General Principles of the Civil Law. In General Principles of the Civil Law, the guardian is for someone "without the capacity for civil conduct." This obviously causes a "cyclic dilemma" in practice. The guardian of a patient cannot be determined if the patient is not identified as having no capacity for civil conduct following legal declaration procedures, which makes it impossible to clarify all people who may assume guardianship as provided in Mental Health Law.

2. Issues in the aspect of providing mental health services (C)

Mental Health Law does not emphasize that mental health services should be as important as physical health services. So, the economic aid and protection of rights for people suffering from mental disorders are obviously different from those for the physically disabled, which is apparently improper.

3. Issues on the rights of people suffering from mental disorders (D)

To start with, a special chapter should be added to Mental Health Law to carry out "protection of the rights for people suffering from mental disorders." Such rights should be protected by law. Some rights (like privacy) are not specific to the recipients of mental health services, but shared by all recipients of health services. However, due to violation of human rights, humiliation, and discrimination for a long time, and sometimes because of the special nature of mental disorders, people suffering from mental disorders may need special and extra protection. Sometimes, people suffering from mental disorders are not treated as adults but as children—even animals. People often think that these people lack decision-making capacity, and thus totally ignore their feelings and dignity of human personality. Many countries (including Brazil, Lithuania, Portugal, Russia, South Africa, the Former Yugoslav Republic of Macedonia, and many other countries) have set, in their mental health laws, specific chapters to provide the rights of people suffering from mental disorders, especially their rights in getting mental health services like the right of communication and visitation, the right to receive education, the leisure and entertainment right, the right to have religious beliefs, etc.[1]

Secondly, a system for informing people suffering from mental disorders of their rights should be established; that is, mental health institutions must inform people suffering from mental disorders of all their rights consistent with the law in the way and language the latter can understand. The above information should also include interpretations of such rights, specific ways of exercising such rights, protests and appeals, and the channels for contact. It can even provide the development of a national pamphlet with unified contents, posters, and videotapes, as well as other ways that are highly understandable and can reflect people's rights (e.g., Statement of Your Rights as Patient issued by the Department of Mental Health and Addiction Services of the State of Connecticut, US, and Instrument on Informing People Suffering from Mental Disorders of Their Rights issued by the State of Maine, US) to fulfill the statutory obligation to keep them informed.[2]

Thirdly, Mental Health Law should pay more attention to the involvement of the public than other health legislation, so it should ensure that recipients of mental health services, family members, or main nursing workers take part in the development of mental health laws and policies and service plans.

---

1   *Resource Book on Mental Health, Human Rights and Legislation* (World Health Organization, 2005).

2   Wang Yue, "History of Protection of the Rights of People with Mental Disorders in the United States and the Successful Experience," *Cross-Strait Legal Science*, no. 2 (2012): 30.

4. Issues in the aspect of the rights of family members and other nursing workers and the agent's decision on treatment (E, K)

Since people suffering from mental disorders generally lack the ability to protect themselves compared with normal people, more efforts should be made to involve their family members and main nursing workers in the development and implementation of patient treatment plans. However, Mental Health Law only provides that medical establishments performing "surgeries that cause internal organs to lose functions" or "experimental clinical care for treatment of mental disorders" shall inform the patient or his guardian of the treatment plan and treatment method, which is apparently likely to be abused. The scope of consent solicitation should be expanded to operations, special body examinations, and special treatment defined in Administrative Regulations on Medical Institutions, and medical institutions should "implement such treatment only after obtaining consent" instead of only giving a "notice."

Mental Health Law fails to set up the Mental Health Care Advance Directive system recommended by WHO. For example, the Mental Health Care Act of the State of Montana, US, provides that the Mental Health Care Advance Directive may be executed by adults with capacity, minors above the age of 16, or minors who are set free, and the above people shall be allowed to make advanced wise and rational prediction of medical decision-making on possible circumstances in the future. "With capacity" here means being able to understand the benefits and risks of healthcare, understand the alternatives to the healthcare to be provided, and understand the communication between the doctor and the patient and make decisions (2011, H.B. No. 518). Besides, after the person loses capacity, he may designate a directive agent to make healthcare decisions on his behalf. If a directive is given when the person does not have the capacity and is irreversible, the agent may make a decision on his behalf in order to protect his client (the person); it is morbidly allowed or legally permitted that the authorized directive agent makes decisions on the event and that the healthcare management provider makes decisions on and records healthcare. The person may wholly or partially, orally or in writing, revoke the directive at any time, unless it is not allowed by the state the person lives in when the person is incapable, or within a certain period after the decision on the incapacity is made. Lastly, healthcare providers will not be punished by the criminal law or civil law for allowing the execution of the directive or the use of such directive before it is revoked.

5. Issues of involuntary hospitalization and treatment (I, J)

To start with, according to WHO legislation proposals, the prerequisite to involuntary hospitalization must include "the purpose of hospitalization is for treatment," which is not clarified in Chinese Mental Health Law, so the purpose of compulsory medical treatment in China is debatable. In particular, there are no effective treatment measures for some special mental disorders like personality disorders in the medical circles now. More importantly, according to Mental Health Law, a person suffering from severe mental illness meets the requirement for involuntary hospitalization when "there is a danger of self-injury, or there is a danger that he will endanger the safety of others," which obviously makes "danger" a reason for hospitalization. Involuntary hospitalization in China is de jure unjustified as a result. Can we find a legal basis to deprive a person who does not suffer from mental disorders yet has the "danger" of killing others of his personal freedom?

Secondly, Mental Health Law does not define any independent authoritative agency to manage such involuntary hospitalization, so it is not in a position to set a time limit for such an authoritative agency to make decisions. Mental Health Law, on the one hand, provides that diagnosis and medical appraisal procedures for a person who suffers from mental disorders and has the "danger of self-injury or danger that he will endanger the safety of others" and is involuntarily admitted can be started again (however, such appraisal must be made under the entrustment of the patient's family instead of an independent authoritative agency), and on the other hand sets the periodic inspection duties of health administrative departments, but fails to clarify whether the patient admitted or his family can complain to the health administrative departments directly.

Thirdly, Mental Health Law fails to differentiate involuntary hospitalization and involuntary treatment, whereas WHO sets different standards on involuntary treatment and involuntary hospitalization in its legislation proposals; that is, involuntary treatment must not be given to a patient who meets the standards for hospitalization, yet is capable of making an independent decision on the treatment he is informed of, or if the treatment cannot improve the patient's physical conditions. Besides, Mental Health Law fails to clarify that involuntary treatment shall be rapid, within a time limit, and checked periodically.

6. Issue of involuntary treatment in the community (L)

Mental Health Law, though mentioning the importance of community treatment, fails to clearly define that involuntary treatment in the community can be an alternative to hospitalization for implementing the principle of "least restrictive treatment."

Principles for the Protection of Persons with Mental Illness and for the Improvement of Mental Health Care (MI Principles) adopted at the UN General Assembly in 1991 has established the principle of treatment in the least restrictive environment, that is, every patient shall have the right to be treated in the least restrictive environment and with the least restrictive or intrusive measures appropriate to the patient's health needs and the need to protect the physical safety of others.[1] Following the principle of the least restrictive alternative, some countries have enacted laws to allow patients to receive involuntary treatment in the community they are living in. The degree of restriction of community facilities is usually thought to be lower than that of hospitals (though highly restrictive living conditions and highly intrusive medical interventions may also be viewed as part of the community treatment order, and they sometimes have a higher degree of restriction than short-term hospitalization). Less restrictive placements usually include outpatient treatment, day hospitalization and treatment, partial hospitalization programs, and family-based treatment. Some countries develop provisions for involuntary treatment in the community for other reasons.[2] There are also countries that have community supervision orders that re-

---

1 UN General Assembly, "*Principles for the Protection of Persons with Mental Illness and for the Improvement of Mental Health* Care," *Principle* 9, no. 1 (1991).

2 K. Harrison, "Patients in the Community," *New Law Journal*, no. 276 (1995): 145; T. Thomas, "Supervision Registers for Mentally Disordered People," *New Law Journal*, no. 145 (1995): 565.

quire patients to reside in designated places and attend specific treatment programs (like consultation, education, and training), and such community supervision orders allow individuals to receive services provided by mental health professionals at home, but not unapproved drug therapies. There are also countries that have issued community treatment orders, including provisions on involuntary drug therapies. New Zealand has revised its mental health legislation following the least restrictive principle. According to Paragraph 2 of Article 28 of the Mental Health (Compulsory Assessment and Treatment) Act, if the court has determined the (involuntary treatment) eligibility criteria, "the court shall make a community treatment order unless the court considers that the patient cannot be treated adequately as an outpatient, in which case the court shall make an inpatient order." Such legislative provisions aim to promote community-based treatment instead of encouraging the outdated system under which patients receive treatment in hospitals. Some countries also introduce the concept of conditional leave according to the least restrictive principle to help patients who have received involuntary treatment in hospitals reintegrate into society.[1]

7. Issue of emergencies (M)

According to Article 29 of Mental Health Law, when a person suspected of having a mental disorder does something to hurt himself or endanger the safety of others, or there is a risk that he will hurt himself or endanger the safety of others, his close relatives, employer or the local public security organ has the legal obligation to deliver him to a medical establishment for mental disorder diagnosis in the event of an emergency. However, in Mental Health Law, there is a limitation, set in reference to WHO legislation proposals, on the time of emergency hospitalization, which shall be no more than 72 hours. Many countries provide that emergency involuntary hospitalization or treatment shall not exceed 72 hours, allowing enough time for completing substantial involuntary procedures of all kinds. For example, Canada

---

1 M. S. Swartz et al., "Can Involuntary Outpatient Commitment Reduce Hospital Recidivism? Findings from a Randomised Trial with Severely Mentally Ill individuals," *American Journal of Psychiatry*, no. 156 (1999): 1968–1975.

provides that, under the premise of respecting the patient, the psychiatrist shall issue a certificate of hospitalization within 24 hours after examining the patient. Such a certificate shall remain valid for 72 hours and shall be regarded as invalid if not implemented within the time limit, in which case the psychiatrist has to reexamine the patient and issue another certificate of hospitalization. The certificate of hospitalization is sufficiently effective, with which mental illness specialists may send the patient to the designated medical institution mandatorily and shall, during the period, take care of, observe, assess, treat, and control the patient for 24 hours. If the psychiatrist taking in the patient fails to issue a new medical certificate within 24 hours, the patient shall no longer be kept by force.[1]

In emergencies, according to WHO legislation proposals, it is strictly prohibited to give patients with mental disorders electric shocks, conduct psychosurgery on them, or take sterilization measures against them, which is not mentioned in Mental Health Law.

8. Issue of special treatment (0)

Mental Health Law does not specifically point out that sterilization or abortion must not be conducted on patients on the grounds of mental illnesses without getting the latter's informed consent, which is very meaningful. Both at home and abroad, there were tragedies that people suffering from mental disorders who might be raped and become pregnant were forced to be sterilized or aborted by their families or the psychiatric hospital.

Article 43 of Mental Health Law requests the patient's or his guardian's written consent only when a medical establishment intends to perform a surgery that may cause an internal organ to lose functions, the scope of application of which is apparently too narrow. Actually, before giving drug therapies to a person with mental disorders or doing surgeries on him, the patient's or his guardian's written consent should be obtained. In the meantime, Mental Heath Law should explicitly provide that doctors shall be allowed to give the patient drug therapy or surgery if the patient's life will be

---

1   Li Dong, "A Comparative Study of the Mental Health Legislation in China and That in Alberta of Canada," *China Health Law*, no. 3 (2012): 19.

endangered in the process of waiting for informed consent. Under normal circumstances, it is a basic requirement that the doctor's general rights are subject to the patient's rights in order to realize patient freedom and autonomy. However, under extremely special circumstances, the patient's autonomy should be restricted, and the doctor's will be realized so as to fulfill the doctor's obligations to the patient and be responsible for the patient's fundamental rights and interests. Such a right is known as Therapeutic Privilege. It exists in many professions, like firefighters and lifeguards.

As regards electroshock, a special therapy with a long history, Mental Health Law totally evades its applied objects and limitations. It should be highlighted in the law that the patient's or his guardian's informed consent must be obtained in order to give the patient treatment of electroshocks. It should be prohibited by the law to conduct non-modified electroshocks on the patient, and clearly forbidden to conduct the electroshock therapy on minors regardless of what mental disorders they are suffering from.

9. Issue of constraints and restrictions (P)

Mental Health Law does not provide a maximum time limit for the implementation of the constraint and protection system, nor does it require a necessary interval after one cycle of constraint, after which constraints and restrictions can be used once more. It may lead to the consequence that constraints and restrictions are abused in practice as a measure to punish people with mental disorders. So when supplementing the above provisions, Mental Health Law should clearly provide that the reasons for each constraint and the time of each constraint must be kept in the medical records completely and truthfully for future reference, and the patient's family members or guardian must be notified that constraint will be imposed on the patient.

10. The supervision and investigation mechanism (R)

Article 50 of Mental Health Law provides that administrative departments of health under people's governments at the county level and above shall periodically review medical establishments in their administrative areas that perform mental disorder diagnosis and treatment. However, it should be clarified in later legislation whether health administrative departments shall launch examination and supervision procedures for separate cases on an ir-regular basis when the patient or his guardian complains about involuntary hospitalization or involuntary treatment, and specific provisions should be developed on the procedures for complaint acceptance, examination, etc. in detail.

Personnel composition of the supervision and investigation agency is of great practical significance, because the hospitalization and treatment of many people suffering from mental disorders is not only a medical issue, but also an issue that involves judgment of values and social tolerance. Hence, besides mental health specialists, there must be lawyers and social repre-sentatives in such agencies. For example, the Mental Health Act of Alberta, Canada, provides that a review panel shall be composed of (1) the chair or a vice-chair (lawyer), (2) a psychiatrist, (3) a physician, and (4) a member of the general public.[1]

11. Issues of police responsibilities and people suffering from mental illnesses and causing accidents or trouble (S, T)

Currently, there are four categories of compulsory medical measures against people suffering from mental illnesses in China. The first category is "com-pulsory medical measures for security," which are specially taken against people with mental disorders who violate Criminal Law and Public Secu-rity Administration Punishments Law. Decisions on admitting such people are made by the public security organ. Ankang Hospitals are psychiatric hospitals or asylums in China which especially admit such people with mental disorders and are under public security organs. "Compulsory med-ical measures for civil relief" fall into the second category. They are taken against homeless people with mental illnesses or demobilized servicemen suffering from mental illnesses. Decisions on admitting such people are made by the civil affairs department. "Family protection-based compulsory medical measures" fall into the third category. The patient's family members, out of paternity or guardianship, entrust a hospital to mandatorily admit the patient suffering from mental illness for medical treatment. It belongs

---

1   Mental Health Act, Revised Statutes of Alberta 2000: 30.31

to the field of civil law, and what is established between the patient's family members and the hospital is a medical service contractual relationship. Such hospitals that admit people suffering from mental disorders belong to the health department. The fourth category is "hospital protection-based compulsory medical measures," that is, where it conforms to the circumstances provided in Subparagraph 2 of Paragraph 2 of Article 30 of Mental Health Law and the patient's guardian hampers hospitalization and treatment or the patient gets separated from hospitalization and treatment without permission, the medical agency may require taking compulsory medical measures against the patient with the assistance of the public security organ. Though the Mental Health Law was formulated by the Standing Committee of the National People's Congress, it fails to clearly define the compulsory medical measures involving people with mental disorders of all kinds in China, and avoids the first and second categories of compulsory medical measures instead. As a matter of fact, people with mental disorders against whom compulsory medical measures of the first and second categories are taken need legislative protection more than people with mental disorders against whom compulsory medical measures of the latter two categories are taken.

12. Issues of the protection of the disadvantaged groups among people with mental disorders (Z)

Mental Health Law fails to provide special legislative protection for children, women, and minorities that are the disadvantaged groups among people with mental disorders, which is to be further improved. Special attention should be paid to the issue of protecting children with mental disorders. It should be made clear in the law only when all feasible community mental health service programs are tried and tested can children with mental disorders be sent to a mental health agency involuntarily. For children patients in mental health agencies, the law must provide that they shall live in an environment independent of that for adult patients and appropriate given their age. All invasive treatment for children against their mental disorders should be prohibited by the law.

Death with Dignity

Death is the inevitable final destination for every living person. As the philosopher Martin Heidegger argues, "Death is being towards death or living towards death."[1] This assertion is one of the catchphrases most often quoted in modern thought but most difficult to understand. Because of the strong influence of feudalism, people in China often think about death only before they die. However, many patients are already completely unconscious before they die, and they have no capacity to think about death. Due to the rapid development of modern medical technology, ventilators and extracorporeal circulation machines have created the hope of prolonging human life, but have presented medical professionals with a dilemma: Is it possible to prolong the process of dying without the use or withdrawal of the life support system, for a large number of terminally ill patients who suffer from incurable diseases and are totally unconscious?

I. Concept of Death with Dignity

The concept of death with dignity is a new term in China, which is easily confused with euthanasia and passive euthanasia. At present, the definition of death with dignity is controversial among scholars in China and abroad. According to Japanese scholar Katsunori Kai, the so-called death with dignity refers to the newly developed life-sustaining technology, which makes

---

1   Martin Heidegger, *Being and Time*, trans. Chen Jiaying and Wang Qingjie (SDX Joint Publishing Company, 2006), 440.

the patient become a medical object, and physicians allow the patient to request to die as the patient refuses the artificial life-sustaining treatment. In
addition to vegetative patients, death with dignity is also applied to patients
with dementia, leukemia, cancer, renal failure, and patients in a vegetative
state.[1] According to Hitoshi Otsuka, a Japanese scholar, death with dignity
is a medical act of removing life-sustaining devices and discontinuing the
prolongation of the life of a patient in a so-called vegetative state who has no
hope of recovering despite the advancement of medical technology.[2] Satoshi
Ueki, a Japanese scholar, believes that death with dignity refers to the in-
terruption or discontinuation of therapeutic practices, and it is the patient's
own decision to stop the meaningless treatment, maintain his or her dignity
as a human being, and face death naturally.[3] According to Japanese scholar
Takehiko Sone, in a narrow sense, death with dignity refers to the termination of life-sustaining measures, such as the removal of a ventilator, for a
patient who has no hope of recovery and is at the end of his or her life. In a
broader sense, death with dignity refers to the termination of special medical measures for patients, including those who have fallen into an irreversible vegetative state.[4] According to Chen Ziping, death with dignity is also
known as "death with elegance" or "natural death." It refers to the measure
of discontinuing futile life-prolonging medical treatments for terminally ill
patients who have no hope of recovering, so as to enable them to face death
in a natural state with human dignity.[5] According to Li Hui, death with
dignity is "euthanasia" for vegetative patients, but it is more appropriately

1   Katsunori Kai, "Death with Dignity from the Perspective of Criminal Law," in *Criminal Law Inquiry*, ed. Liu Mingxiang and Tian Hongjie, trans. Ren Jihong (People's Public Security University of China Press, 2008), 57–60.

2   Hitoshi Otsuka, *Outline of Criminal Law*, trans. Feng Jun (China Renmin University Press, 2003), 360–367.

3   Satoshi Ueki, *Medical Jurisprudence*, trans. Leng Luosheng et al. (Law Press China, 2006), 357.

4   Takehiko Sone, *An Introduction to Criminal Law*, trans. Li Hong (Law Press China, 2005), 79–80.

5   Chen Zhiping, "The Effects of Euthanasia and Death with Dignity in Criminal Law," *The Latest Legal Document Interpretation*, no. 6 (2007).

called "death in peace."[1] Zhang Mingkai argues that advances in medicine have made it possible for vegetative patients to sustain their lives by relying on certain devices. Death with dignity describes the act of removing a life-sustaining device from a vegetative patient.[2]

As far as the above scholars' definitions of death with dignity are concerned, the main difference lies in the two aspects of the object of application of death with dignity and the way of its implementation. With regard to the object of application of death with dignity, except for Satoshi Ueki, who has not explicitly limited it, scholars' views are divided into the following four categories: First, as Katsunori Kai argues, death with dignity has the broadest scope of application and refers to patients who are incurable, including, for example, patients with senile dementia. Second, as Chen Ziping argues, death with dignity is limited to patients who are at the end of their lives and cannot be recovered. Third, Hitoshi Otsuka and Zhang Mingkai are conservative and limit the application of death with dignity to vegetative patients only. Takehiko Sone and Li Hui, on the other hand, hold the fourth argument that death with dignity only applies to patients in a vegetative state who have fallen into an irreversible state of unconsciousness. In the author's opinion, the first view apparently enlarges the scope of those to whom death with dignity applies. It would be inhumane to extend the scope of death with dignity to those who suffer from diseases without effective curative treatments. The second view emphasizes that the patient is at the end of life, but does not stress that the patient must be unconscious, so it is less rigorous. The third view is limited to vegetative patients. However, it is ignored that even vegetative patients may awake again, and even healing miracles may occur. The fourth view defines the application of death with dignity to end-of-life vegetative patients who have fallen into an irreversible state of unconsciousness, and it is relatively rigorous.

Regarding the implementation of death with dignity, scholars mainly disagree on whether the termination of artificial medical measures includes

---

1   Li Hui, "Commentary on the Types of Euthanasia," *Journal of Shanghai University of Political Science Law (The Rule of Law Forum)*, no. 2 (2011).

2   Zhang Mingkai, *Outline of Foreign Criminal Laws* (Tsinghua University Press, 1999), 148–187.

nutrition and water replenishment. Scholars in favor of the termination of nutrition and water replenishment argue that nutrition and water replenishment can be terminated because they are artificial medical acts. Minoru Otani, a Japanese scholar, also argues that the termination of nutritional supplementation, such as stopping nasal cannulae or stopping intravenous fluids, is an artificial act of active medical treatment. Therefore, depending on the patient's condition, it is considered to be possible to stop such supplementation.[1] A similar view was expressed in the Report of the Special Committee on Death and Medical Treatment on Death with Dignity, published by the Academic Conference of the Japanese Medical Association. The negative view is that all artificial medical treatment can be terminated, but nutrition and water replenishment must be maintained. Once the nutrition and water replenishment is stopped, the patient may not die because of the disease, but rather starve to death because of the lack of nutrition and water replenishment. The author agrees with the latter viewpoint, because it is not inevitable to remove the artificial respirator and the artificial dialysis machine and simply supply nutrients and water to the patient. Still, it may allow the patient to be dignified before the end of his life. If the former view is adopted, the patient will have no dignity, not to mention the natural outcome of the disease.

To summarize, the author believes that death with dignity implies that all active medical interventions to sustain the life of a vegetative patient who has fallen into an irreversible unconscious state at the end of life are removed, so that the patient can die naturally and with dignity.

---

1 Minoru Otani, *An Overview of Criminal Law*, trans. Li Hong (Law Press China, 2003), 203–204.

II. Death with Dignity and Euthanasia

1. Death with dignity and euthanasia

The term euthanasia is derived from the Greek word "euthanasia," meaning mercy killing, the act or practice of painlessly putting to death. In *The Oxford Companion to Law*, euthanasia is described as the causing or hastening of death for patients, especially at the request of a patient suffering from an incurable disease or a critical illness.[1] According to Ni Zhengmao, euthanasia means that a dying patient who is unable to endure physical pain has his/her life ended as painlessly as possible by a physician at his/her request and in accordance with legal procedures. Voluntary consent is required to commit euthanasia.[2] Qiu Renzong argues that euthanasia is the intentional causing of a person's death as part of the provision of medical treatment to that person.[3] Scholars' description of euthanasia can basically be summarized as a humane way for physicians to end the life of a patient who is suffering from an incurable disease in a painless state. At first glance, death with dignity is no different from euthanasia. Some scholars even equate death with dignity with euthanasia in their studies of euthanasia, arguing that death with dignity is an alternative name for euthanasia. Death with dignity and euthanasia are also confused in the legislation and discussions in many countries and regions. However, there are essential differences between the two. Mixing the two is not conducive to the protection of the rights and interests of terminally ill patients. More importantly, people's fear of euthanasia may not be conducive to the promotion of the system of death with dignity and the establishment of a general social consensus. Death with dignity differs from euthanasia in the following aspects.

---

1   David M. Walker, *The Oxford Companion to Law*, trans. Li Shuangyuan, et al. (Law Press China, 2003), 399.

2   Ni Zhengmao, Li Hui, and Yang Tongdan, *Research on Euthanasia Law* (Law Press China, 2005), 39.

3   Qiu Renzong, *Bioethics* (China Renmin University Press, 2010), 135.

First of all, the objects of application are different. Death with dignity only applies to vegetative patients who have fallen into an irreversible status of unconsciousness at the end of their lives. In contrast, the objects of the application of euthanasia are broader than those of death with dignity, and it applies to all patients at the end of their lives. Second, the application motives differ. Both the requests for death with dignity and euthanasia have the same motive of alleviating pain, but the sources of pain are different. Patients requesting death with dignity are already vegetative patients in an unconscious state, suffering no physical pain, and their motives for requesting death with dignity are mainly the huge economic and mental burden on their families. The motive of euthanasia request is that the patient cannot bear the huge pain in the body. Third, the purpose of implementation is different. Death with dignity advocates following the laws of life and embracing death naturally, which is a way to "optimize" the quality of life. Euthanasia, on the other hand, is an artificial and intentional interference with life. It is an "abandonment" of life, not a natural death. Fourth, the applicants are different. Euthanasia must be initiated voluntarily by the patient when he or she is conscious. Death with dignity is usually applied by a close relative of the patient when the patient is unconscious. Fifth, the time to death is different. Death with dignity takes place in a sedate manner, such as by removing the ventilator. As a result, the time to death is not very certain after its implementation, and it generally progresses slowly. Therefore, death with dignity is easily accepted by the general public. Euthanasia, on the other hand, is administered in a hasty manner, such as by the injection of a lethal drug. Hence, the time to death after euthanasia is defined, and it often progresses rapidly. For this reason, euthanasia is less likely to be accepted by society and ethics. Sixth, the stage of dying is different. In medical research, experts usually divide the development of the death process into three stages: agonal, clinical, and biological. Patients who opt for death with dignity are in the agonal stage in medical terms, whereas those who opt for euthanasia, although suffering from incurable diseases, are not in the agonal stage in medical terms.

2. Death with dignity and passive euthanasia

Some scholars have suggested that death with dignity is equivalent to passive euthanasia. Based on the way how euthanasia is performed, it is divided
into active euthanasia and passive euthanasia. Active euthanasia means
taking certain measures to hasten the patient's death, which is sometimes
known as aggressive euthanasia. Passive euthanasia refers to discontinuing
measures to sustain the patient's life and leaving him or her to die.[1] Passive
euthanasia refers to discontinuing measures to sustain the patient's life and
leaving him or her to die.[2] James Rachels, an American scholar, holds a different view, arguing that there is no clear-cut distinction between active and
passive euthanasia.[3] The distinction between active and passive euthanasia
has no moral relevance to euthanasia, as both are cases of death, not means
to death.[4] In fact, there is no difference between active and passive, positive
and negative, or active and inactive euthanasia. The withdrawal of a ventilator from a terminally ill patient may seem passive, but it is an active act. It
may seem passive, but it is also aggressive. It seems to be a way of inaction,
but it is also a way of action.

In the author's opinion, the classification of euthanasia into active
euthanasia and passive euthanasia according to the mode of execution is
indeed questionable, and it may be more appropriate to classify euthanasia
into slow euthanasia and rapid euthanasia according to the progress of
dying. Even if the classification of active and passive euthanasia is adhered
to, death with dignity and passive euthanasia are the same concept because
of the different targets.

1 Xu Zongliang, Liu Xueli, and Zhai Xiaomin, *Bioethics* (Shanghai People's Publishing
   House, 2002), 258.
2 Ye Li, "An Exploration of the Legalization of Death with Dignity" (Hunan University,
   2010), 4.
3 James Rachels, "Active and Passive Euthanasia," in *Biomedical Ethics*, ed. T. Mappe and J.
   Zembaty (NY, McGraw Hill, 1981).
4 Ronald Munson, *Intervention and Reflection: Basic Issues in Bioethics (I)*, trans. Lin Xia
   (Capital Normal University Press, 2010), 301.

III. Analysis of the Decriminalization of Death with Dignity

1. Analysis of decriminalization of death with dignity from the perspective of grounds of justification

As a key concept in the civil law system, grounds of justification refer to the grounds that exclude the illegality of an act that conforms to the constituent elements. Generally speaking, a behavior that constitutes a crime in civil law countries needs to be evaluated from both positive and negative sides. From the positive aspect, the conditions for the existence of a crime are the conformity of the constituent elements, the unlawfulness, and the culpability of the act. Any act that objectively conforms to the constituent elements is considered to qualify as a constituent element. Although, in principle, an act conforming to the elements is unlawful, there are exceptions to this rule. That is to say, in the case of special reasons and grounds, it may also deny the unlawfulness of the behavior that meets the constitutive elements. It is the grounds of justification, also known as "grounds of exclusion of crime."[1] As the basic content of the theory system of grounds of justification, three doctrines exist in civil law and criminal law (the doctrine of superior legal interest, the doctrine of soziale adäquanz, and the doctrine of purpose). The following is a decriminalization analysis of death with dignity, using the rationale of these three doctrines.

> Doctrine of superior legal interest

Originating from the doctrine of legal interest measurement, the doctrine of superior legal interest holds that the actor should assess and weigh the harm and benefit of the legal interest of the act before performing an act. If the benefit of the legal interest of the act is assessed and weighed to be greater than the harm to the legal interest, the act can be regarded as having grounds for justification. Given that death with dignity is preceded by a true expression of the will of a particular patient, it assesses and weighs the

---

1   Zhang Mingkai, *Outline of Foreign Criminal Laws* (Tsinghua University Press, 1999), 148.

patient's own interests and the interests of the patient's family. First of all, when compared horizontally with other people's interests, the patient's own interests appear to be "superior legal interest." Secondly, when compared vertically with the interests of life, the patient's interest in a high quality of life is also a "superior legal interest." Generally, we consider the self-interest of each individual in his or her own life as the supreme legal interest. However, when an individual is dying and has little chance of recovery, and his or her body can no longer deliver any benefit to the individual, the value and social significance of the life will be dramatically diminished. The patient defaults to a diminished interest in his or her own life, and it is replaced by what the patient believes to be the best interest of his or her life, which is consistent with the principle of humanity that the law seeks to achieve. One of the functions of criminal law is to safeguard human rights, so that the vast majority of people in a country can live a happy life.[1]

> *Doctrine of soziale adäquanz*

The doctrine of soziale adäquanz holds that the illegality of an act should not be determined solely on the basis of whether the legal interests have been impaired or not, but rather on the basis of a specific and comprehensive analysis of the behavioral pattern and its value. A judgment should be made as to whether it is an act of social adequacy. Only acts that deviate from social adequacy are illegal. The doctrine of soziale adäquanz takes social identity formed on the basis of the history of the society in which the act is committed, customs, and habits as the basis for judging whether or not the act is illegal. Death with dignity is a manifestation of people's pursuit of quality of life and the value of life. For this reason, it carries a noble humanistic spirit. From the point of view of social development, the concern for the population's quality of life and the population's quality represents a leap forward in the progress of human society and a reality that cannot be avoided. Secondly, from the viewpoint of social resource conservation and sustainability, death with dignity is considered appropriate for the development of the present society and even more so for the future society. Accord-

---

1   Cesare Bonesana Beccaria, *On Crimes and Punishment*, tans. Graeme R. Newman and Pietro Marongie (New Jersey: New Brunswick, 2009).

ing to a report by the Ministry of Health, Welfare, and Family of Korea in 2009, "A Study of People's Opinions on Stopping Life-Sustaining Treatments and Legalization Programs," 93% of more than 1,000 interviewees agreed with treatment such as the removal of ventilators for patients with terminal cancer.[1] Thus, it can be seen that death with dignity is an act of social adequacy, and the changing attitudes of the population indicate that death with dignity is increasingly permitted by the ethical process. Death with dignity manifests an advanced perception of the development of things and is in compliance with the law of the end of life.

> ***Doctrine of purpose***

The doctrine of purpose holds that the act of the actor constitutes a contravention of the law because the act conforms to the "common purpose of life" recognized by the state, i.e., the stability of the social order. Without a stable social order, the common life of society must not be guaranteed accordingly. When considering the issue of death with dignity, we should not rigidly apply the provisions of the criminal law, but should examine it from the perspective of the legal order and the spirit of the law. Death with dignity is obviously not contrary to the Constitution of the People's Republic of China, because the death with dignity of the citizens accords exactly with the respect and protection of human rights. Patients may choose the option of death with dignity by means of Living Will or Power of Attorney of the durable power of attorney, which is a normal and proper exercise of the citizens' rights. Then, the execution of death with dignity by a physician for a patient demonstrates respect for the exercise of the rights of others, and death with dignity does not violate the basic spirit of civil law. On the contrary, death with dignity can be regarded as a special civil contract established between physicians and patients. It also represents the significance of the basic principles of "freedom of contract" and "autonomy of will" in civil law. Therefore, it can be seen that the physician's implementation of death

---

1   Ye Li and Chen Ce, "The Legitimacy of Death with Dignity from the Grounds of Justification of Civil Law System," *Journal of Changsha Railway University (Social Science Edition)*, no. 2 (2010).

with dignity for the patient, both in terms of form and essence, is not in violation of the relevant provisions of Chinese laws.

2. Analysis of the decriminalization of death with dignity from the theory of anticipated possibility

Anticipated possibility is a theory of the actor's subjective aspect (culpability) proposed by scholars who advocate normative theories of culpability. It refers to the possibility that the actor can be expected to perform a lawful act under the specific circumstances at the time of the action. By contrast, unanticipated possibility means that in the specific circumstances of the act, it is impossible to expect him to perform any other lawful act than the criminal act in question.[1] Hobbes supposes that a person is compelled to commit an unlawful act out of fear of immediate loss of life, or a person is in want of food or other necessaries of life and has no other alternative to preserve himself except by committing a crime, as if he had robbed or stolen in a famine when he was unable to pay for any food with money or receive it in charity. Then that person may be fully forgiven, since no law may bind a person to forsake his efforts to preserve himself.[2]

Throughout all the judgments on euthanasia cases handled by Chinese judicial organs, the anticipated possibility has never been addressed. Does it mean that China's judiciary does not recognize the theory of anticipated possibility and its specific functions in individual cases? No. The theory of anticipated possibility is characterized by the evaluative meaning of "ubergesetzliches." The theory of anticipated possibility has been replaced by another term in China, or is dominating the basic ideology of criminal trials in China in another legal capacity. This term is "social harmfulness." In the case of euthanasia in Hanzhong, Shaanxi, the key reason why the client was ultimately exempted from punishment was that his actions were "not socially harmful, and he committed a minor offense." According to the theory of anticipated possibility, the law can only require people to do what they

---

1   Liu Renwen, "Crisis Theory in Criminal Law," Institute of Law, http://www. iolaw. org. cn/ shownews. aspid=1164.

2   Thomas Hobbes, *Leviathan*, trans. Li Sifu et al. (The Commercial Press, 1985), 234–235.

are likely to do and cannot force them to do what they may not be able to do. If we need to confirm that the perpetrator is indeed guilty of the act, we must be able to anticipate that the perpetrator will commit a lawful act rather than an unlawful act in the light of the specific circumstances at the time of the act. Unanticipated possibility involves two situations. One is where objective conditions render the perpetrator completely incapable of deciding autonomously on his own conduct. That is, the conduct he commits is the only choice he can make. The other is that the perpetrator may choose to commit a lawful or unlawful act. If a lawful act is taken, the perpetrator's own interests may suffer significant damage.

For death with dignity, the patient must be suffering from an illness that is considered incurable by contemporary medicine. In this case, the patient has two options. On the one hand, the patient may choose to die naturally, continuing hopeless treatment and bearing a huge financial burden. On the other hand, they may choose to die with dignity, to end their lives with dignity and in a humane way. It is worth noting that whichever option is chosen, it is merely a matter of time before the patient dies. As a result, there is no deprivation of the patient's right to life. In this case, death with dignity, for both the patient and his family, is a last resort when the patient's consciousness is in a normal state, and his violation of the regulations is a forced act. If there is no such compelling situation, the perpetrator will not consider committing such a violation of norms. Thus, death with dignity is the only option. If a patient on the verge of death suffers from a terminal illness, or if a relative or friend of the patient makes a sincere request to let the patient die with dignity without violating the patient's will, the physician may perform the necessary procedures of diagnosis and consultation before letting the patient die with dignity, out of compassion to terminate or end the patient's life and to let the patient die in a humane and dignified manner. In such cases, the judge may make an empirical judgment based on the empathy and common sense shared by the general public of the community when faced with the same circumstances. If it is considered not to be reasonably anticipated that a physician would be indifferent to a terminally ill patient who is incurably ill and in extreme pain, the basis of culpability of the physician may be excluded, and the physician may not be convicted. In this way, the death with dignity can be de facto decriminalized. The theory of anticipated possibility to explain death with dignity is premised on the basic consideration that the law does not force people to do anything that they are not willing to do, and that the law respects and sympathizes with the weaknesses of human nature.

IV. Cases and Legislation on Death with Dignity in Some Countries and Regions

1. Cases

The Karen Ann Quinlan case is an important milestone for death with dignity in the United States. Karen Ann Quinlan has been in a coma since 1966 when she drank a cocktail at the age of 12. She was on a ventilator to keep her heart beating and on an IV drip to support her nutrition. She was 21 years old in 1975. Her father requested to be her guardian. As a guardian, he had the right to consent to the withdrawal of all medical treatments, including the removal of the ventilator. The High Court of New Jersey rejected his claim, holding that "to approve of this would be to kill the girl" and that it violated the right to life. The Supreme Court of New Jersey, however, reversed the High Court's decision and granted the father guardianship over his daughter, allowing him to withdraw all medical treatment with his daughter's physicians. The Karen Ann Quinlan case was unprecedented in US history because the court permitted the patient's family to remove the patient's ventilator.[1]

In 1980, US citizen Brother Fox was sustained by a ventilator in a vegetative state. He had previously verbalized his desire to follow Pope Pius XII's advice not to be sustained by "extraordinary means" if he were in a condition similar to Karen Ann Quinlan's. The New York State Court of Appeals concluded that Fox had a right of customary law to refuse treatment. This right to refuse treatment remains in place after the patient is incapacitated,

---

1   Qiu Renzong, *Bioethics* (China Renmin University Press, 2010), 123–124.

as long as there is "clear and convincing evidence that he has expressed a desire to do so.[1]

In 1983, Nancy Cruzan, a US citizen, had a car accident in Missouri that left her in a vegetative state. Convinced that their daughter had no chance of regaining consciousness, Nancy's parents petitioned the court to remove her artificial feeding and watering devices and allow her to die naturally. Since Nancy's parents could not present written proof of their daughter's intent to refuse treatment, the Supreme Court of Missouri denied Nancy's parents' request, pursuant to the Missouri Living Will Statute, which specifies that "a citizen has the right to refuse medical treatment, but only if his or her consent is expressed in writing."[2]

In February 2008, a 75-year-old Korean woman, Ms. Kim, suddenly suffered a ruptured blood vessel and massive hemorrhage when she underwent a bronchoscopy in the hospital for suspected lung cancer. She fell into a coma due to hypoxia in her brain and became a vegetative patient. And ever since, she had been supported in the intensive care unit by a ventilator and a feeding tube. After the hospital refused to remove the ventilator, Ms. Kim's children filed a lawsuit for death with dignity in the court on their own behalf and behalf of their mother. They requested the termination of the meaningless treatment of their mother. On May 21, 2009, the Supreme Court of Korea ruled in favor of removing Ms. Kim's life-sustaining device based on the provisions of the Constitution, which stipulate that "the patient shall have the right to decide on or change his or her treatment."[3] It is the first time that a Korean court has ruled that the will of a vegetative patient can be respected to discontinue unhelpful life-prolonging treatments and allow the patient to meet his/her death naturally.

---

1   Qiu Renzong, *Bioethics* (China Renmin University Press, 2010), 123–124.

2   Matsui Shigenori, "On the Right to Self-Determination," trans. Mo Jihong, *Foreign Law Translation and Review*, no. 3 (1996).

3   Anonymous, "Korea's Grand Court Approves 'Death with Dignity' for the First Time," *Global Rule of Law*, no. 6 (2009).

2. Legislation

> *United States*

The Karen Ann Quinlan case led to a national awareness of death with dignity in the US. In 1976, the Natural Death Act was enacted in California, making it the first law in the world on "death with dignity." The Natural Death Act emphasized the application of death with dignity by providing that "any adult may, in a conscious state, leave a copy of the Living Will in advance." The purpose of "Living Will" is to allow patients who have no hope of recovery to express their will in a document in advance before they lose their judgment. Moreover, under specific circumstances, the patient's attorney may be legally authorized to act in accordance with the patient's will, including directives to forgo medical treatment. Currently, most states in the United States have enacted natural death acts or legislation on death with dignity that is equivalent to such an act.

> *Germany*

In June 1986, Germany enacted the Act on Assisted Dying, which contains specific provisions for safeguarding the human dignity of terminally ill patients. Among them, Article 214 (1) stipulates the circumstances under which a patient's life support device can be withdrawn. Subparagraph 2 provides that a doctor who interrupts or controls treatment on the basis of the patient's true will may not be subject to a penalty. Influenced by the American system of living will, some German civil organizations have strongly advocated the introduction of this system, with only a slight difference in the names, such as the statement of the patient's will.[1]

> *Japan*

On May 26, 1994, the Academic Conference of the Japanese Medical Association published a Report of the Special Committee on Death and Medical Treatment on Death with Dignity. In the report, the conditions for termination of life-prolonging medical treatment are stated as follows: "If the

---

1   Shu-Yu Tseng, *Medicine, Law, and Ethics* (Angle Publishing Co., Ltd, 2007), 204–205.

patient is in a state that is medically unlikely to recover, and it is deemed to be more than a vegetative state; if the patient expresses his/her will to accept death with dignity when he/she has the capacity to do so, and the will may be withdrawn at any time. The act of termination of life-prolonging medical treatment should be performed by the physician in charge as a measure based on medical judgment, and it should preferably be done with the consent of the patient's near relatives."[1] Although death with dignity has not been recognized in Japan by legislation so far, adults are allowed to enter into a "Living Will" in writing. For example, in Japan, the Association for Death with Dignity was spontaneously established to advocate living will to the general public. The will indicates that "if my illness is incurable by current medical treatments, and I am diagnosed to be on the verge of death, I will refuse all unnecessary attempts to prolong my life." However, the Japanese government is cautious about this, and so far, there is no legislation on "death with dignity."[2]

> **Singapore**

In 1996, Singapore enacted the Advance Medical Directive Act, and it came into force in July 1997. The Act provides that any Singaporean citizen of 21 years of age or above who is conscious and capable may sign an advance directive in the presence of two persons of full civil capacity, one of whom shall be a medical practitioner. The medical practitioner shall assist the person concerned in executing the provisions of the advance directive to fulfill the patient's will when the conditions are satisfied.[3]

> **Taiwan, China**

In June 2000, Taiwan, China formulated and adopted the Regulations on Hospice and Palliative Care. Hospice and palliative care refers to the provision of palliative, supportive medical care or the withholding of cardio-

---

1   Anonymous, "Reflections on the Concept of Death with Dignity," *Contemporary Medicine*, no. 9 (1995).

2   Ye Li, "An Exploration of the Legalization of Death with Dignity" (Hunan University, 2010), 4.

3   Luo Diandian, *Who Decides When I Die* (The Writers' Publishing House, 2011), 18.

pulmonary resuscitation (CPR) in order to alleviate or relieve the pain and suffering of a terminally ill patient. The regulations apply to terminally ill patients, i.e., those who have suffered from serious injuries or illnesses diagnosed by a physician as incurable and for whom there is medical evidence that the course of the disease will progress to the point where death is unavoidable in the near future. In Taiwan, terminally ill patients are required to make a "letter of wishes" to choose hospice and palliative care. The person who wishes to do so may appoint an attorney for medical care in advance and specify the purpose of the appointment in writing. When the person is incapable of expressing his or her wishes, the proxy may sign on his or her behalf. At any time, the person may withdraw his/her wishes in writing, either by himself/herself or by his/her attorney.

V. Vision for the Institutionalization of Death with Dignity in China

1. Application for death with dignity

The scope of applicants for death with dignity should be all natural persons with full capacity for conduct. If the application for death with dignity is considered to be prudent, it can also be moderately limited. For example, the Regulations on Hospice and Palliative Care in Taiwan stipulates that only those over 20 years of age with full capacity for conduct are allowed to make a letter of wishes in advance.

The way of expressing the intent of death with dignity and the way of applying for death with dignity can be addressed by referring to the ways of advance directives, living will, and durable power of attorney that have been gradually introduced in Europe and the United States in the past decade or so. These ways were created out of concern that in the event of a critical illness or sudden accident, the person concerned may not be able to express his or her will because he or she may become unconscious. At present, there is no provision for "Living Will" in the legislation of mainland China. However, the efforts made by some civil organizations on death with dignity have contributed to the development of death with dignity objectively. For example, in May 2009, the "Choice and Dignity" public welfare website published Five Wishes, the first folk text suggested for use in mainland China. Specifically, the five wishes are "The person I want to make healthcare decisions for me when I can't make them for myself," "The kind of medical treatment I want or don't want," "How I Want People to Treat Me," "What I Want My Loved Ones to Know," and "How Comfortable I Want to Be." It hopes that by promoting Five Wishes, more people will be aware of what a Living Will is and how they can use it to anticipate and handle the risks they may encounter at the end of their lives. It should be noted that the Five Wishes, similar to "living will," offered on the website "Choice and Dignity," do not have any legal effect. The activities of such non-governmental organizations are more about educating and informing people about death. The lack of identification on the Internet makes their activities hardly feasible in practice.

Singapore's Advance Medical Directive Act stipulates that advance directives shall be attached to the patient's medical file. Medical personnel are only allowed to inquire whether a patient has signed an advance directive if the patient is in a coma. The United States law specifies that all public hospitals and nursing homes shall be informed of whether or not a patient has signed an advance directive when the patient is admitted to the hospital. Due to China's special national conditions, a "multi-track parallel model" should be implemented at present. That is to say, legislation should be passed to require eligible citizens to register their will to die with dignity when applying for a driver's license, registering for national health insurance, or registering for a patient's medical record upon admission to a hospital. The specific application method can be any one of the options of advance directives, living will, and durable power of attorney. Citizens should also be allowed and encouraged to hand over these legal instruments to their family members or friends.

In the Nancy Cruzan case, Sandra Day O'Connor, justice of the Supreme Court of the United States, made the important point that for most people, rather than making a will before they die detailing how they should die of natural causes without resorting to medical treatment for sustaining their lives, it would be better for them to entrust someone, who could be a loved relative or a close friend, to make the decision for them in such a situation. She argued that the Constitution granted people the right to choose to die. However, she also emphasized that the Supreme Court's decision denying

Cruzan's parents' request did not violate this right, since Cruzan herself had not made a formal power of attorney. It is especially important to note that the Power of Attorney (which is similar in nature to the durable power of attorney), which is used in practice by medical institutions in China, takes an implied approach to the selection of specific therapeutic options for a patient in a coma. That is, it only informs the patient in writing that the specific therapeutic regimens are to be chosen by the attorney if the patient is unconscious, but it does not expressly state that the specific regimens include waiver of resuscitation. Such a Power of Attorney does not have the legal effect of empowering the attorney to decide on the death with dignity for the patient. Regarding the choice of death with dignity, an express statement of intent must be made, regardless of which of the options of advance directives, living will, and durable power of attorney is taken. An implied statement of intent should be invalidated.

If the patient for death with dignity has never made any kind of written application for death with dignity during his or her lifetime, who can decide on his or her behalf whether to sustain or terminate his or her life? This question is premised on the difficulty of identifying the will of the patient and the fear that the right to death with dignity may be abused. From the basic concept of the right to life, life is inalienable and non-transferable. However, in the course of social development, people have left part of their autonomy over life to be governed by the state or society. If a vegetative patient who has suffered a severe traumatic brain injury and is in a coma or unconscious state is unable to express his or her wishes in an unconscious or incapacitated state, his or her family members or physicians have little or no way of knowing whether or not the patient is willing to have his or her life terminated prematurely. Is it possible to simplify the dilemma of this situation by saying "maybe"? Such a hasty presumption of consent is plainly mistaken. In the case of Nancy Cruzan, the Supreme Court of Missouri abrogated the lower court's judgment on the ground that Cruzan's parents did not have "clear and convincing evidence" that the termination of medical treatment was the personal will of Cruzan, who was in a vegetative state. Cruzan's friend testified that in a conversation after Cruzan's grandmother passed away, she heard Cruzan mention that she preferred death to live as a zombie. However, the Supreme Court of Missouri ruled that this testimony could not constitute sufficiently strong evidence to warrant a permissive ruling (the Supreme Court of the Federal Government still upheld the decision of the Supreme Court of Missouri by a vote of 5 to 4). Although the Supreme Court of the Federal Government denied Cruzan's parents' request, it upheld the general constitutional right of persons with capacity, which means that they have the right to decide not to accept medical technology to sustain their lives.

2. Judgment of death with dignity

The court is the judicial organ of a country and a symbol of its judicial authority, and its decisions are authoritative and conclusive. It is most appropriate for the court to verify the application for death with dignity. Under the simplified procedure, the court may examine the relevant advance directives for death with dignity, the "Living Will," the "Power of Attorney" of durable power of attorney, and the medical certificate from a medical practitioner that the patient has fallen into an irreversible vegetative state. Upon confirmation, the court should issue a notice granting execution of death with dignity, and the specific time and place of execution of death with dignity and the relevant procedures should be indicated in the notice. In order to facilitate management, the judiciary should establish a comprehensive system of files on death with dignity. The content of the file should comprise the patient's basic information, advance directives, living will, power of attorney, and the medical certificate issued by the medical practitioner that the patient has fallen into an irrecoverable state of health.

3. Implementation of death with dignity

After obtaining a written notice from the court permitting the execution of death with dignity, the executing personnel must execute the death with dignity in strict accordance with the legal procedures. Prior to the operation, the local procuratorate should dispatch an officer to witness and supervise the operation and notify a representative of the family to be present. The hospital staff should make a written record of the execution of death with dignity. The record should be signed or stamped by all participants, witnesses, and supervisors and submitted to the People's Court for further reference. The execution of death with dignity should be done by a qualified physician for vegetative patients who are in an irreversible state of unconsciousness at the end of their lives. It is mainly implemented by terminating all artificial medical treatments, including termination of blood transfusion, medication, cardiopulmonary resuscitation, artificial chemotherapy, artificial dialysis, artificial ventilator, cardiac pacemaker, and other artificial medical treatments, as well as nutritional and water replenishment.

4. Supervision of death with dignity

Supervision of death with dignity begins with judicial supervision. When death with dignity is carried out, the court may notify the local public procuratorate to dispatch an officer to the scene to supervise the execution of death with dignity and ensure that it is conducted strictly with the established procedures. Secondly, there is industrial supervision. The medical association of the patient's place of residence should supervise the implementation of death with dignity, including technical supervision on whether the patient is in an irreversibly unconscious and vegetative state at the end of life. It is recommended that death with dignity should be implemented only after a consensus is obtained between the hospital physicians and the medical association experts. Thirdly, there should be social supervision. Data on the implementation of death with dignity should be made available to the public to prevent abuse of power and trampling of life.